ENDINGS & BEGINNINGS

ENDINGS &
BEGINNINGS

Sandra Hayward
Albertson

RANDOM HOUSE NEW YORK

*Grateful acknowledgment is made to the following for permission to reprint previously
published material:*

The Hogarth Press Ltd. and W. W. Norton & Company, Inc.: The lines from "The
Tenth Elegy" are reprinted from *Duino Elegies* by Rainer Maria Rilke, translated by
J. B. Leishman and Stephen Spender, with the permission of W. W. Norton &
Company, Inc. Copyright 1939 by W. W. Norton & Company, Inc. Copyright
renewed 1967 by Stephen Spender and J. B. Leishman. Acknowledgment is also made
to St. John's College, Oxford Translators and The Hogarth Press Ltd for permission
to reprint the above material.

Random House, Inc.: Excerpts from "The Bear" are reprinted from *Go Down, Moses*
by Willian Faulkner. Copyright 1940, 1941, 1942 by William Faulkner. Copyright
1942 by The Curtis Publishing Company. Copyright renewed 1968, 1969, 1970 by
Estelle Faulkner and Jill Faulkner Summers. Reprinted by permission of Random
House, Inc.

Library of Congress Cataloging in Publication Data
Albertson, Sandra Hayward.
Endings and beginnings.
1. Albertson, Sandra Hayward. 2. Albertson, Mark.
3. Christian life—Friend authors. 4. Death.
5. Consolation. 6. Terminal care. 7. Lymphoma—
Biography. I. Title.
BX7795.A48A33   248.8′6   79-4769
ISBN 0-394-50627-8

Manufactured in the United States of America
24689753
First Edition

For Robin and Kim

Blessed are they that mourn for they shall be comforted.
—Matthew 5:4

They that sow in tears shall reap in joy.
He that goeth forth and weepeth, bearing precious seed, shall doubt-less come again with rejoicing, bringing his sheaves with him.
—Psalms 126:5–6

ACKNOWLEDGMENTS

I owe special thanks to my parents, Betty and Ducky Hayward,
to Mark's mother, Evelyn Lewis Albertson,
to Rebecca Haley McCall,
Barbara McClarin Bing,
and Ruth Bryant Purtilo,
for their invaluable counsel and support;

and to all those friends and family, named and unnamed,
who held us then and since.

CONTENTS

Part I

REMEMBRANCE

CHAPTER
1
Endings and Beginnings

This wasn't the way we'd planned it at all. Mark hadn't wanted to go back into the hospital, ever; he'd so clearly wished to die at home. We'd expected to have all the necessary equipment on hand there: the aspirator, the oxygen unit—everything to make the ending as comfortable as possible—but none of it had been delivered yet. It all happened so quickly—the pain, the sudden weakness, the frightening struggle for breath. We knew that lymphatic cancer often meant death by suffocation. Was this to be it now, so soon? Could one know all along and still be caught so off-guard—ready, but never really ready? Mark had said now, calling the shots as he had all along, "I've got to have some help, San. Let's get me to the hospital."

Here we were once again, this time on the seventh floor, the hospital's resuscitation unit. Mark's bed was wheeled into a stark, antiseptic room, with no pictures or curtains and only a brick-wall view—the very setting we'd been so determined to avoid. I was thrust back into a corner, and the medical staff went to work.

A nurse came with her forms and charts to ask me for Mark's medical history, all the proper admission procedure that we'd by-passed in the emergency room. "And your husband's initial symptoms, Mrs. Albertson?" Where were all the records from Mark's other hospitalizations? What earthly good were they if they weren't used at times like these? Mike, the young physician and friend who'd come with us, saw my despair, took the nurse aside and gave her whatever information she needed.

Mark was barely conscious. His face was without color; his feet were ice-cold. Fluid drawn from his chest revealed internal bleeding, and efforts were being made to hook him up to transfusions. Blood was spattered over the walls and floor. His veins and arteries were in such bad shape from all the chemotherapy injections that the doctors were having a hard time finding an adequate connection.

I stood at the end of the bed, useless, extraneous. Was there nothing anymore that I could do? Would Mark die now, surrounded by doctors and nurses, while those of us who loved him hovered silently in the background?

An anesthesiologist was finally called in, and a suitable connection was made through the jugular vein in Mark's neck. Dr. G. came by and explained that since Mark was hemorrhaging internally, they were going to use transfusions to counter the loss of blood. The internal bleeding accounted for Mark's weakness and difficulty in breathing, his inability to retain oxygen, and the chest pains of the previous night, when some artery must have broken. Unless the bleeding itself stopped, however, the pressure on his lungs would lead to suffocation.

Out of my own anguish, I asked, "What's the point in doing all this? Can't we just let him go without all the heroics and apparatus?" The last thing both Mark and I wanted was for him to be merely kept alive by mechanical means, and Dr. G. knew it.

He seemed startled by my question, and tried to assure me that the transfusions ought to at least be tried. When I asked how long we would have, G. replied only that we would know within the next twelve hours whether the transfusions had been successful. I knew by the way he said it that if the bleeding continued, there would be little time left.

When the catheter had been secured and the transfusions begun, the fervor in the room subsided. Color rushed back into Mark's body; his breathing became more regular, and he was able to talk. I know now that if we had remained at home Mark would have died within a few hours, and that, unequipped as we were to ease his suffering, it might have been a desperate encounter with death for us all.

Time collapses in strange ways during a crisis; suppertime had come and gone. At some point I'd called our Quaker friend Sylvie, and she went to take care of the children so Mark's mother could come in to the hospital. I struggled with whether to call my parents yet. How could I ask them to make the trip again unless it really was the end this time for Mark? I finally told them that although Mark was back in the hospital, there was a chance the transfusions would work and things would be okay for a while longer. They said they'd come regardless, and left within the hour to make the eight-hour journey through the rainy night.

By ten o'clock that evening, Mark was much more himself, uncomfortable and irritated by all the tubes, but not in pain. The transfusions were discontinued. We'd bought some time at least, and had entered another "meanwhile"; all we could do now was wait. I needed to breast-feed my infant daughter Kim, so I went to ask the doctor in charge how he thought Mark was doing, and if it might be all right for me to go home for a little while.

The resident was in his late twenties, about the same age as Mark. He swallowed hard at my question, and replied, "Your husband's demise is not imminent, Mrs. Albertson." I almost laughed, I was so startled by such language from a peer. I said, "You mean Mark's not going to die in the next few hours?" I told him what we knew of Mark's kind of cancer and what Dr. G. had said about the transfusions. We agreed that I was to be notified immediately if Mark had difficulty breathing or began to get worse in any way. I asked Mark if he would mind my going, and when he said he'd be okay, I left him with his mother for the night.

I don't remember how I got home. Someone was there to take me —probably Mike, who was simply and quietly available to help in whatever way was needed. I realized later that that week was supposed to have been Mike's vacation between hospital residencies and that he and his family had been going to take a trip. When Mark became so much worse, Mike and his wife Vicki had simply decided to use their vacation time for us.

When I got home, Kim was asleep. I made a few phone calls to let friends know what was happening, and Sylvie and I sat up talking. We spoke little of Mark or the hospital. The anguish of that afternoon seemed far away. At home now, it was possible to believe again that it was too soon for Mark to die; to say, "Death, yes, sometime—but not yet."

At six in the morning, the phone rang. It was Ken Sheppard, Mark's high school friend from New York, calling from Mark's hospital room. When he'd learned, through a convoluted chain of phone calls, that Mark had been readmitted, he'd taken a midnight train, arriving at the hospital about 3 A.M. He'd found Mark's room, and relieving Mom Albertson so she could get some rest, spent the early morning hours at Mark's bedside. He was calling now to say that Mark was having difficulty breathing again.

My parents had arrived during the night. I woke them now and my father said he'd drive me to the hospital. Suddenly I didn't know what to wear—a small thing, really, yet it filled me with an aching awareness of last things. My mother suggested my old dungarees and work shirt, knowing how comfortable and how much a part of our life style they were. Since both children were still asleep, I asked Sylvie to bring Kim to the hospital and try to sneak her into Mark's room as soon as she woke.

I waited outside while my father dressed. It was still early, and very quiet—a serenely fresh, rain-cleaned May morning. I was filled with tense expectancy. What would this day hold for us, for all of us? What endings and beginnings? There was so little time left now, and I needed to be with Mark.

I gathered some lilacs from a neighbor's yard to add to the apple blossoms a friend had brought to the house. Just as Dad and I were getting into the car, a mail truck drove up with a special delivery letter for Mark; it was from Becky, our very dear friend in Boston, arriving now, incredibly, just in time.

The streets were deserted; the city barely stirring—a hushed expectancy about the day itself. It felt as it did to me as a child going to an Easter sunrise service. I entered the empty lobby and quiet corridors of the hospital, struggling for inner control.

Mark was awake. I climbed onto the bed and we held each other for a while. Though we didn't speak openly then of what it meant, his breathing was clearly more labored. The phone rang. It was Sylvie on the hospital line downstairs, letting us know that she'd arrived with a very hungry Kim. I met them at the elevator, Sylvie's six-foot frame wrapped in a wonderfully big poncho, Kim hidden inside. My father ran interference with the nursing station, and we squirreled Kim into Mark's room. The young resident on duty came in a few minutes later and said, "On this floor, with intensive care especially, this shouldn't happen, but I think you ought to do it anyway."

Mark lay watching us in the gentle quiet of the morning, and as I nursed our daughter by his bedside, there was for us a deep sense of the continuity of life. When Kim had finished, Mark laid his hand on her little head in an unspoken blessing, and she was tucked back under Sylvie's poncho for the trip home. They'd just turned the corner when the nursing supervisor came in for her early morning rounds.

What satisfaction we derived from that transcending of a hospital rule, yet how trapped we still were by hospital policy. I do not comfortably break rules, and except for those times when we took Robin, our three-year-old, up to the tenth-floor lounge, and once to a private room, I'd been successfully cowed by the NO VISITORS UNDER 14 sign. There was no reason now, however, for any age restriction on visitors to Mark's room. There was no disease a child might transmit that would have harmed Mark any further. Yet I did not break the rule again to send for Robin to see her father one last time.

Mark must have known that things were getting worse. Mike arrived and Mark said to me, "San, let's get me out of here and home while there's still some dignity left to me." He asked Mike if he'd be able to be with him and willing to administer morphine at the end, knowing that morphine would both relieve the pain and make the letting-go process easier. Mike said he would do whatever he could to help, and went to ask Dr. G. about getting Mark discharged.

Mike returned to say that if going home was what Mark wanted most it could be done, but he explained how difficult the return trip itself might be, and what toll it would take on whatever strength Mark had left. Mark had always said he wanted to know the truth about his body, if he had only a few days to live, he did not want to waste those days. It was time now to honor that trust. Holding his hands in mine, I told him then that his difficulty breathing probably meant that we had less than twelve hours left together. He was quiet for a while, and then said that if it was okay with me, he'd not try to get back home again.

Dr. G. came into the room soon afterward. With dignity and a knowing mind, Mark asked him to "pull the plugs" so that he could die without the heroics. "My God, Mark, I can't commit euthanasia," G. replied, and turned and walked out. I wondered then if Dr. G. would honor Mark's desire to die on his own terms, according to his own internal timetable.

A nurse appeared in the doorway. She explained that Dr. G. had just ordered all previous medications stopped and had assigned her to us for the day. She asked to be told anything that would help her to be of help to us as a family. She said she would be working throughout the ward, but would be immediately available to us whenever we needed her. We never did call for her specifically, but I was grateful for her sensitivity, for her own risk-taking, as well as for that gesture on Dr. G.'s part, an official sanctioning of human caring on the part of the medical staff.

While I was still in the corridor, Dr. G. came by and explained that they would do another chest tap to give Mark some relief in breathing and then would begin administering morphine. I was relieved that it was to be as Mark had wished, and said I'd let Mark know about the morphine right away. "Don't tell him about it," exclaimed Dr. G. "There's no reason not to," I replied. "It's what Mark has asked all along to have happen at the end."

My anger and despair at the medical world the day before for taking over the care of the person I loved was not to last. Care for Mark now took on a new form. The emphasis was no longer on treatment and recovery, but on physical comfort and support.

When the resident had completed the chest tap and was removing the needle, Mark said to him, "While you're at it, why don't you just take out the rest of this stuff." Without a word, the resident undid the IV tubes in Mark's arm, and within seconds removed the needles and mass of tape from his neck which the anesthesiologist had labored so to insert the night before. Mark was freed. He could turn his head as he wished; no tubes constricted his movements now, no needles or tape dangled off his body. An aide came in and washed the blood off the walls and floor and took away all the apparatus for administering transfusions. The only medical equipment that remained was a nasal oxygen unit inserted in the wall which Mark could choose to use or not to help his breathing. There was a real sense of living just in that moment, of being present where we were.

A nurse brought supplies for giving Mark a bath. I asked if I could do it, and she left us alone. Bathing this body, wasted and battered now by its struggle against an unremitting foe, was a last loving act for me to perform. It was, I suppose, rather like the ritual of preparing the body that family members themselves used to do prior to burial. When the bath was finished and the bed changed, the nurse came to give the first shot of morphine, and Mark slept.

At some point that morning, I asked Mike Earnest if he would do whatever else was necessary to complete arrangements for the corneal transplant and the donating of Mark's body to the hospital's medical school. The forms that Mark and I had sent for earlier from the State Anatomical Gift Board still needed the witnessing of final signatures, something we'd never gotten around to doing—a part of the psyche's delay mechanism, I suppose. Although as next of kin, I could make the final arrangements after his death, I took the forms to Mark now. I asked him if he was still clear about his wish to give his body for medical research, and if he wished to sign the authorization himself. He was, and did, with a last painful but determined signature.

As the day progressed, Mark slept off and on. I began reading to him from Sigurd Olson's *The Singing Wilderness*. The opening paragraph described the loons of the northern wilderness lake country where the author had traveled by canoe, reminding us of a canoe trip in Maine when we, too, had seen our first loons. It felt now as if we had come full circle.

I also read Becky's special delivery letter, a warm reaffirming of Mark's importance in her life and of her continued holding of us. While I was looking at the morning newspaper, Mark noticed an ad promoting Mother's Day, two weeks off. He never did give exotic gifts, and there was no big "last gift" gesture on his part now. He'd been planning to get his mother a splatter shield for cooking fried foods, and he asked if I'd take care of it for him.

Sylvie came in again, without Kim this time, and offered to massage Mark's feet. They were joking about whether there were thirty-four or thirty-six metatarsal bones when Dr. G. came to the doorway to ask Mark how he was feeling. Mark replied that his most pressing problem at the moment was accounting for the number of bones in his foot, and Dr. G. threw up his arms in mock dismay and went on his way.

From time to time I brought Mark the lilacs and apple blossoms to smell, though much of the day was spent just being quietly present. There was no sense of needing to speak much—no sense of having unfinished business. That, at least, was the result of being open during these last four months. We had already done some of the grieving together, had shared tears and talked about the problems.

Later, as the doses of morphine took cumulative effect, Mark began to hallucinate and rock from side to side in the bed. Much of what he said we couldn't understand, although he explained his thoughts at great length, with careful attention to detail. At one point, knowing that I didn't really understand him, he said, "Thanks for listening anyway." Though I was grateful for the easing of his pain, I missed being in touch with him during those times.

Mark talked about the songs that we'd sung with Rob and Becky, about some of the special ones they'd written for him. Then, of all the songs he knew, he proceeded to sing one about a prune: "No matter how young a prune may be, he's always full of wrinkles; a baby prune is like his dad; he's just wrinkled half as bad." He spoke intently about a new planet which had been discovered recently beyond Jupiter, and then of the amazing symmetry of our three-year-old's drawings. He gave a rambling but detailed description of the texture of whole-wheat bread, a kind I often made for our family and one which he knew was to be a central part of his memorial celebration.

My mother had been caring for the children at home, but she came into the hospital in the late afternoon, knowing that it was probably the last time she would see Mark. She offered to wash his hands, a last loving act. She's said since that whenever she washes her grandchildren's hands she thinks of their father, the image of his slender fingers mirrored in theirs. Mom used that time to tell Mark again that he was loved as a son-in-law and a part of their family. There were no theatrics or teary goodbyes, simply the affirming of their love for him and the place he held in their lives.

When Mark and his own mother were alone for a few minutes, he turned to her and said, "Well, Mom, I guess there's not much left to say." She told him she wished she could take his place, but he replied, "It's still a pretty nice world." She thanked him now for what he had meant to her for those twenty-nine years, and for what he had given her —a loving daughter-in-law and two beautiful grandchildren.

I'd been dreading the time when Mark might choose to withdraw from those around him, might need to be free from our need of him, our grief. It was not to be that way this day, at least not for us. In the midst of incoherent ramblings, he startled us by recognizing and greeting Charlie, his closest friend among the graduate students, who'd just arrived from an afternoon class. Other friends were gathered in the corridor outside the room and Mark called out, "Where is everybody? Bring the party in here."

Later, as I sat alone with him for a while, Mark's rocking became more agitated, his murmuring more troubled. He kept repeating, "Too young, too young." Then he began to thrash about wildly, as if trying to get out of the bed. His breathing became gagged and desperate. I tried to hold him back, but had to summon the nurse. Mike and several nurses came running. They helped get the side rails up and held Mark down. The sound of his breathing was so awful and the rush of medical attention such a contrast to the day's earlier calm, that I thought this was the end. Then, as suddenly as it began, the thrashing subsided, and Mark became quiet.

The afternoon turned to dusk, Mark dozing, rocking again, alternating between ramblings and clearness. Dr. G. came in and asked, "How are you doing, old boy, any pain?" Mark nodded yes, which startled me since he'd not complained, and none of us had thought to ask. Dr. G. patted Mark on the shoulder and left, a nurse returning immediately with pain medication. Dr. G. did not come in again; he was not with us at the end. But he had respected Mark's wishes to exit as he had asked, and for us that day, it was enough.

Mark commented calmly at one point that his vision had become double. Mike explained that it was an effect of the medication rather than the tumor itself. The two friends talked quietly, Mike gently explaining the medical processes that were taking place as Mark's body neared death.

Suddenly Mom Albertson realized that Mark was trying to say something, that he was asking for something to drink. He'd taken no solids and only a few liquids in the last forty-eight hours. Now he drank a great deal of ginger ale, and to our amazement, asked for some of the brownies that Vicki had sent in with Mike that morning. It was the first solid food he'd showed interest in for days. The brownies were divided, and along with the glass of ginger ale, shared with everyone in the room.

Breathing became more and more difficult for Mark. He spoke little, except to ask the time—as if taking final measure of the day left to him. He rocked back and forth, his lips touching my hand. Then, as he struggled to lift his head, his mother said, "He wants to be kissed." My own numbness at this point had missed those simple signals, and I bent at last to respond. He said then, "Let's call it quits, okay, Pooh?" and I replied, "Yes, if you can go in peace."

It was nearly seven now; the hospital was quiet. Time seemed to hang in a balance, as if undecided about proceeding. Mark's condition remained the same; waiting was now the most difficult part. I got up, at last, to stretch my legs, and went with a few others to the lounge at the end of the corridor. We'd been gone only a few minutes when Ken came running up the hall urging me to come quickly.

Several nurses and a woman resident were in the room. Mark was thrashing about again, as he had done earlier, struggling for breath. I sat on the edge of the bed, holding on to one of his hands. Soon the thrashing ceased, and in the silence that followed I said, "Go in peace, Pooh." Charlie turned to Ken, standing beside him at the end of the bed, and asked if it would be all right if they took hands, that it would feel better that way. Our friends around the bedside held each other while we waited.

I found it hard to look at Mark's face then. It was drained of color, and a paralysis of his facial muscles gave him a distorted, unfamiliar appearance. It was not to be an easy death, no gentle slipping into sleep. Mom Albertson has said how peaceful she remembers him looking when it was all over, and I am glad for that.

The doctor continued to listen to Mark's heart, and when she indicated that he was still alive, Mark's mother said, "Mark, we love you very much." A few moments later, the doctor removed her stethoscope and closed his eyes.

My father held me and kept saying, "Go ahead and cry, it's okay to cry." But I had no tears. I hadn't begun to know my own pain yet. Right then, in that place and at the end of that struggle, death seemed appropriate, understandable, even acceptable. It was clear to me that Mark's spirit was no longer there; it was an empty shell that remained on the bed. For me there was only an immediate glad acceptance that he had been released from physical suffering, and freed to go a new and different way.

A nurse offered to bring us some tea, and we sat in the corridor outside the room, drained, yet relieved that it was over—released, now, ourselves.

The cornea must be removed within a few hours of death, and a doctor from the eye bank had been standing by. When he'd finished, a nurse asked if we wished to return to the room. I said I didn't. Quite frankly, I didn't want to see what had happened to Mark's eyes. (I know now that there would have been no visible evidence of the medical procedure.) Besides, I'd already said goodbye, and there didn't seem to be any point in prolonging the ending. We all held each other once more, and then went our separate ways.

Robin was awake when I arrived home, waiting for me to kiss her good night. I took her in my arms, and told her that Mark had died. I explained that in spite of all that the doctors had tried to do, his body had been too sick to continue living, and that his pain was over now. I told her that her dad had loved us all very much, that he had not wanted to die, and that it wasn't anyone's fault. I had to tell her that he would not come home again, ever, and that like other living things that died, his body would be buried in the ground, would be returned to nourish the earth. Then I told her that all that had been good and true and special about her dad would never really end, that we would remember his love for us, and would continue to be held in his caring.

Robin's tears did not come immediately either. I held her for a while in the quiet darkness, and then tucked her into bed.

CHAPTER
2
Beginnings
of an Ending

It was a special night out for Mark and me, a festive break before exams began for him the next week. The University Glee Club's Christmas program opened with Randall Thompson's "Last Words of David"; we did not know that evening that last things had begun for us as well. When Mark leaned across a railing during intermission to speak to a friend, I was startled to see him recoil with pain. It signaled to me for the first time that his recent stomach discomfort might not be just a case of nervous tension before exams. He'd been sweating a lot at night lately, yet his temperature remained normal and there didn't seem to be anything really wrong. His abdomen had become somewhat bloated looking over the past month, but we'd just joked about his sympathetic pregnancy—I was expecting our second child in six weeks.

Mark had never been one to pamper his body; he usually couldn't even be persuaded to take an aspirin for an occasional headache. He'd always kept himself in good physical shape, this past year bicycling the fifteen blocks from our apartment to the University of Pennsylvania each day. That his stomach should be a bother now, just as final exams were starting, puzzled and irritated him. Finally, the day before his first exam, Mark went to the student health clinic. The doctor on duty didn't examine him, but prescribed some Maalox for his nervous stomach.

I'm glad, in a way, that Mark's illness was not discovered then, for it meant that we were able to have a big family Christmas together as planned. Mark got through his exams, which completed his graduate course work in computer science and left the winter semester clear for writing his master's thesis and attending to his teaching assistantship responsibilities.

The night before we were to leave for Christmas vacation at my parents' home, Mark's sweating was worse than ever, which seemed odd now that exams were over. His temperature was normal the next morning, so we gathered up Robin, Mark's mother, a student friend, the dog, Christmas presents, projects and snow gear, and headed off for New England.

Our families have always tried to get together at Christmastime— grandparents, children, in-laws on all sides—taking turns at each other's homes. This year there were thirteen of us, including my twin sister, Sue, her husband, David, and their children, who came on from Chicago. We were to go up to Vermont later to spend some time with my older sister's family, since they couldn't leave their dairy farm.

It was a good Christmas gathering, full of the excitement of children, the delight of homemade gifts, good food, long stories, old jokes and deep laughter. We cut down our own Christmas tree, a balsam, romped in the snow, and took turns preparing meals, everything from roast beef to black bean soup. Oliver Powell, David's father, the minister who'd married Mark and me, and a dear friend as well, read *A Child's Christmas in Wales* by Dylan Thomas. We delighted again in the account of an old Welsh Christmas; like the dog in Dylan's verse, ours got sick on the rug.

It was still clear, however, that Mark was not well. Sweat covered his brow almost constantly now, and though he did not speak of it, others noticed that he was not himself. His nights continued to be troubled and restless. When he could not sleep, I got up with him and we talked into the early morning hours about future plans—about his desire to teach computer science in a liberal arts college setting.

Urged by those around him, Mark made an appointment with my parents' doctor for the day after Christmas. Some friends from out of town stopped in for a visit just before he left for the doctor's—a brief meeting with Mark that was to be their last. When he returned from the appointment, Mark quietly announced that the doctor suspected something was quite wrong and advised that we return to Philadelphia to admit him to the university hospital as soon as possible.

My immediate reaction was disappointment that our vacation was going to be interrupted, that we would have to miss the wedding of friends a few days later, and that this special time with my family was to be cut short.

How naïve I was; how unscarred I was then by any of the tragedy that touches the human condition. Oh, to be sure, I'd seen pain around me, or at least thought I had. I'd lived and worked in the inner city, had spent time in the rural South, had served in the Peace Corps in a developing nation. Whatever ugliness or suffering I'd been exposed to, however, was never really mine. I could put it behind me whenever I chose.

In almost seven years of marriage, neither Mark nor I had really been sick. We both did lots of outdoor physical things: bicycling, camping, backpacking. Neither of us smoked; we had an occasional beer and drank wine with special dinners. We ate a balanced diet (the "proper" one green/one yellow vegetable), meatless meals once a week, and home-made bread.

We left my parents' home the following morning, assured of the loving concern of the whole family, yet confident that all would be cleared up shortly. Mark drove the whole eight-hour journey home; I was the one who was irritable, uncomfortably eight-months pregnant and occupied with the traveling antics of our three-year-old.

Mark's mother returned with us, and asked to stay until his medical problem was at least clarified. She was much more anxious about Mark at this point than I. His father had died on an operating table two years earlier, and Mark was her only child.

The next morning, Mark took the trolley in to the student health clinic for another checkup. He returned at noon to say that he was to be admitted to the hospital within the hour. Another doctor had confirmed that something was indeed quite wrong and suggested that exploratory surgery might be necessary.

I was stunned. I rushed about gathering things for Mark's hospital stay, yet was conscious of my own helplessness. There was something dreadfully empty and futile about packing a toothbrush and pajamas to send the person I loved to the hospital. It suddenly occurred to me that he wouldn't be home that night, and I began already to know a sense of loss.

There were hurried hugs with Robin, who was puzzled yet comforted by our assurances of Mark's return. This time I drove Mark to the hospital. We walked in from the parking lot, savoring now that time alone together. Along the way, Mark noticed a forsythia bush, trying in the late December thaw to send out some buds. He grinned, seeing in it a good omen.

Various tests were begun on Mark, but the New Year weekend arrived and everything except emergency cases was set aside. Mark was given a six-hour pass to spend at home during each day of the long weekend. Though it was good for us to have him at home, it was hard on Mark. He was obviously sick; his features were strained, and his abdomen increasingly distended. When he asked to get back to the hospital after only three hours on Sunday, I knew we'd just been pretending that things were all right. While he read Robin one last story, I got out the camera and took a picture of them, with a sudden sense of the fleetingness of that scene. Photography, a hobby then for Mark, was to become for me a conscious attempt to capture certain moments, a way of claiming the essential image of a relationship whose temporal dimensions were to become all too obvious.

No one doctor was assigned yet to Mark's case. Because it was a teaching hospital connected with the University of Pennsylvania what Mark did receive was lots of attention from great bands of medical students. They would gather around the bed, examining, prodding, repeating procedures and questions. Mark was sure that every student available practiced their proctoscopy on him.

Numerous questions were asked about our Peace Corps experience in East Africa six years earlier—the climate we'd lived in, the elevations we'd climbed to, the kinds of persons with whom we'd been in contact, and the medical problems to which we'd been exposed. With that emphasis during the examinations and questioning, Mark and I supposed that he had some tropical disease. It all seemed rather adventurous and dramatic, but certainly not life-threatening. The tests went on for ten days. We were told only that the results were inconclusive.

Robin wanted to see Mark, and we managed it for a while by sneaking her up to the tenth-floor lounge for patients and visitors. How forbidding were those hospital signs prohibiting the visiting of young children, and how difficult for young families. Robin and Mark's need for each other was far greater at this point than any risk from childhood diseases.

It had always been a part of our family routine for Mark to read Robin a story at bedtime. The first time I took Robin into the hospital, she waited for him in the lounge hallway with her little face aglow. When he stepped off the elevator, however, she could only exclaim, "Daddy's in his pajamas!" It took some explaining, for she was not to see an actual hospital room for some time. For several evenings Mark and Robin read stories and did puzzles together. Then the evening came when Mark had to use a wheelchair to come to the lounge, and had such difficulty breathing that he could not finish the story which Robin had brought. He soon became too weak to leave his bed, and Robin's visits came to an end.

Mom Albertson stayed on in our apartment, waiting with us for some change in Mark's condition, and helping to care for Robin whenever I was with Mark in the hospital. When she returned to her own home at one point to check on things, she was gone overnight, leaving me alone with Robin for the first time since Christmas. It was the day for the garbage cans to be taken out to the front sidewalk, a task Mark usually performed for our whole apartment building. As I dragged the cans out to the edge of the curb, I had a fleeting thought that Mark might never again be there to carry the trash out, that he might never come home again at all. Overwhelmed with a sense of loss I stood among the garbage cans, tears streaming down my face. Back inside, for the first time in a long time, I prayed—not for cures or miracles, but for strength —for all of us.

During that first week and a half of tests and questioning, it seemed as if nothing was being done to ease Mark's suffering or to keep him from getting worse. His sweating was constant and severe. My resentment grew at what seemed to me to be inadequate nursing care for the simple provision of comfort. His bedding and pajamas were frequently soaked, and at last we were supplied with some absorbent pads that could be more easily changed. At least those physical acts of caring—assaulting the laundry room, securing linens for Mark's bed, even the ritual at home of preparing fresh pajamas—gave Mom Albertson and me something to do, easing the tension which surrounded these days.

The dynamics of hospital roommates and their families is a story in itself. There were numerous changes during Mark's own stay, but several of the patients made lasting impressions as they became caught up in each other's medical dilemmas. When one fellow needed respiratory exercises, the physical therapist got the whole room to encourage and work with him. One of the roommates was in terminal stages of lung cancer, and we all waited tenderly with him until the doctors could do nothing more and his family took him home. Though he died a short time later, his brother and sister-in-law stayed in touch with us, visiting Mark even at home and bringing food and toys for the children.

Another patient had made the decision to undergo complicated open-heart surgery rather than live with the constant possibility of heart failure. His courage and will to live and his philosophy about the quality rather than the quantity of life were props for the rest of us, and we all rejoiced when he made it through the risky ten-hour surgery.

There always are, of course, those roommates and visitors that one would not choose to live with—the self-appointed medical experts, the smokers, the whiners, and the TV addicts, but on the whole there is much to be said for the phenomenon of the four-person room. In spite of little in common in our backgrounds, there was genuine concern among the relatives and families of the patients. Trips to the cafeteria, offers of rides home or at least escorts to the parking lots after visiting hours were what we could offer one another.

The medical decision to do exploratory surgery after ten days of tests was a relief to us, as we were sure that it would at last define the problem. We were still confident that once the doctors were able to identify the problem, a medical solution would follow.

The experience of Dad Albertson's death from complications following surgery two years earlier, however, did at least make clear to us the need to take care of some unfinished business before the operation. I asked a lawyer friend for the simplest possible wording for a will in our state, and typed up a three-sentence document for both Mark and myself. It seemed like an appropriate time for me to make a will as well, especially since I would be having Caesarean-section surgery the following month. Friends from our Quaker Meeting came to the hospital as witnesses while Mark and I each signed the wills. Our choice of witnesses made it, for us, more than just a legal act. It was a solemn occasion, and we tried to make it less so by joking about it.

Mark had already met the surgeon on the case, but I had not, since his medical rounds took place early in the day. We both felt it important

that I be included in the presurgery discussions, and Mark had explained
to the surgeon that I would be coming in early the morning before the
operation, specifically to meet him. Mark told me he wanted the surgeon
to know that he wished to be told the truth, whatever the surgical
findings.

During early morning grand rounds, the surgeon arrived with his
entourage of students, typical of a teaching hospital. Dr. C. was charm-
ing to me, and managed the whole exchange with finesse. The medical
procedures were confidently and quickly explained, with a relaxed and
sophisticated humor. The surgery itself seemed to be a routine matter.
Then they all turned and moved briskly out of the room. There'd been
no chance allowed for any personal patient-physician involvement. The
"bedside manner" that had so consciously set us at ease had been at the
expense of real integrity of relationship. Mark and I looked at each other
with a kind of stunned awareness; we had not had a chance to voice any
of our anxieties or express our concern for the truth following the
surgery. Sheepishly admitting that we'd been overwhelmed by the con-
viviality of it all, we chose, in our innocence, to believe that it didn't
really matter. I wonder now what the surgeon and the medical students,
many of them Mark's age, must have been thinking or feeling as they
swept in and out of the room, for we learned later that the surgery itself
merely confirmed what the medical staff already suspected.

I had called my mother and asked if she could be with us during
Mark's operation. I was aware of Mark's mother's anxiety and knew that
my mother's steadfastness and inner strength were what I needed now.
She came, traveling the four hundred miles by bus from Worcester,
Massachusetts, arriving in an unfamiliar section of the city. Lou, an old
friend of Mark's, learned of my mother's travel plans, dashed off to meet
her bus and brought her to our home. Another friend, Vicki, had asked
if she could take care of Robin the day of the surgery. I was grateful and
continually amazed at the creative ways in which we were supported and
cared for by our friends.

The night before the operation, Mark and I talked about the future.
I had been wrestling out my own theological stance on personal suffering, and said to Mark then that regardless of what happened, I did not
believe that there was any divine willing of this crisis for us. Those who

spoke of "God's will" offered no comfort to me at all. Mark agreed, though he was not much for theological wrestlings. He was basically an agnostic with a questing spirit, one who at least kept the doors open, never letting either his own belief or his own doubt interfere with another's questing. It was that openness within our marriage that allowed me to be actively involved in Quakerism and personal spiritual journeying.

The morning of the operation I went into the hospital early. I found Mark already strapped onto the stretcher, ready to be taken to the surgical floor. Though he'd already been given some medication, he was still alert. The nurse handed me his wedding ring, which he had asked that I hold during the surgery. As we touched, I know we were both aware that Mom and Dad Albertson had their last moments together at just such a time two years before. I left him then and joined our mothers in the waiting room.

It was, for reasons all too obvious later, a short operation. Within the hour, I was startled to hear the surgeon speak my name. He had come directly to the waiting room, still in surgical dress. As I stood to meet him he said, "I'm afraid the news is not good." He explained that they had found a tumor in the abdominal cavity which could not be removed surgically. Then he went on to say that they needed to wait now for the biopsy reports before they could determine what kind of tumor it was and what treatment would be most effective. He explained that it was possible that the growth was a form of Burkitt's tumor, common to the East African countries where we had been, and that it could be successfully controlled by X-ray treatment. While it usually appeared in the jaw or neck area in Africans, he said that perhaps it had taken an abdominal form in a Caucasian. That seemed like a strangely unscientific statement to me even then.

It's clear to me now that I did not really hear the doctor say that it was not good news. He probably had no intention of letting that be the thrust of his report to me that day anyway; the fact that I was eight months pregnant probably tempered his presentation of the truth. I do not fault the surgeon for the way he handled his announcement that day. I heard the half-truth that I wanted to hear. I can honestly say that the thought of cancer never crossed my mind, and I had no conscious understanding that a tumor could be terminal.

Both mothers were quietly supportive. We left the waiting room, reassuring each other of the hopeful possibilities, none of us admitting our fear for all that had been left unsaid. Yet when I called my twin sister in Chicago, I suddenly found it hard to tell her that the tumor was inoperable. There was something in the verbalization of that fact that began to make it more real to me. Behind closed doors in the ladies' room, I did some dry sobbing, but there was no release for my feelings yet. Without acknowledgment of the extent of Mark's illness, there was no occasion for an honest response; I had not yet been freed to cry.

The two mothers and I walked across the campus to get some lunch. The tension was even greater now than before; the unknowns even more oppressive. Our very composure was suffocating, and we spoke of soup and trivia.

I returned to sit by Mark's bedside, as he had asked me to do while he came out of the anesthesia. Simply being present helped my own need. When he finally woke, I spoke only of the need to wait for the biopsy results.

That evening, as I left the hospital elevator with a group of young doctors and interns, I was startled to have the head resident surgeon under Dr. C. turn to me and say, "Try not to worry; we'll do everything we can." It was clear there was much more going on than any of us was admitting.

CHAPTER
3
Games
and Covenants

Now the game began. As we waited for the biopsy results, Mark's condition grew steadily worse. He sweated continuously and profusely, and was always thirsty. His breathing became more labored; his eyes, dull and listless. Exactly how much Mark himself knew of the nature of his illness, I am not sure. There is much that I would ask him now if I could. He must have been aware of something. What distorted the whole process was our trust in the medical world.

Mark was told by the surgeon a few days after the operation that it had revealed a lymphatic growth in his abdomen, but that final diagnosis could not be made until the biopsy results were complete. Mark's only comment to me was "Well, if it's lymphatic, at least it's not cancerous." Since Mark was the physicist, the scientist in our household, I assumed that that deduction was correct, that the tumor was not cancerous.

So the waiting continued, this time for the biopsy results, each of us trying to mask our anxiety. We all made attempts at being cheerful, and Mark spoke of getting home before long. In many ways it was easier to be with him in the hospital than to be at home where his absence was real and I could allow myself some thoughts about the seriousness of his illness.

I have always found it hard to keep things in; I find sharing of news is a way of diffusing the weight of it. My phone calls to friends increased in direct proportion to the seriousness of the message. I *had* to talk to others about what was happening to us, all the more because Mark and I were not talking about it to each other. I was able to tell members of our Quaker Meeting about my own anxiety, and even verbalized the possibility that Mark's illness might be terminal. I was able to cry openly with these friends and was, in turn, held and supported by their love and caring. The quality of support between friends and myself was, at that stage, on a deeper level than between Mark and me, and because of that, our relationship itself was less whole. Our trust in each other was being undermined, even violated, by a "protective silence."

Why this conspiracy of silence? To keep his spirits up? or ours? We never made any conscious decision *not* to talk with Mark about the seriousness of his illness. I certainly fell into the pattern of making some casual excuse to leave Mark's bedside and go out after a doctor's visit to learn what had not been said in Mark's presence.

It was, without question, the most difficult time of all for me. Excluding Mark from knowing whatever limited information the doctors were giving me was foreign; the pretense and furtiveness was demeaning, to me and to our marriage. I was keeping something from the person most dear to me. And it was *his* body, *his* future, that we were being so secretive about. Integrity had always been so central to our marriage, that the inability, the failure to share this area of our life together now only intensified my anguish. We continued to wait out the days for the pathology results, as if, somehow, the arrival of new facts would be the essential criteria for deciding whether or not to share the truth.

Mark became increasingly debilitated. No treatment to combat the tumor had yet been initiated. Usually so resilient and strong spirited, he became more and more depressed and withdrawn, either hallucinating or irritable and hard to please.

I finally took in a small "thought for the day," drawn from II Timothy 1: 6–7, and quietly taped it to the side of Mark's bedtable. My mother had sent it, explaining that it had meant a lot to her when my father had been critically ill many years before. I do not usually feel comfortable distributing Scriptural pronouncements, but I did know then that Mark's spirit, as well as my own, needed nurturing.

Hence I remind you to rekindle the gift of God that is within you . . . for God did not give us a spirit of timidity, but a spirit of power and love and self-control.

I was aware of many good people waiting on the sidelines who wished to share their love and concern with Mark, but who remained silent or absent or merely cheerful visitors because of the façade we were all maintaining. Masking the truth meant masking our love. It was, ironically, our "protective silence" that was working to deny Mark any sense of the love and the power or self-control of which II Timothy speaks.

The day before the lab results were due, I felt the need to clear some ground with the surgeon. I made an appointment to talk with him in his office and arrived, feeling very apprehensive, with three main concerns. Mark was eating virtually nothing, yet no one seemed to care. I asked Dr. C. if protein couldn't be made available to Mark in liquid form, and he immediately wrote a memo for the dietary staff. Then I asked him to come in alone and talk to us when the lab report results came in, instead of meeting me in the corridor or arriving with all of his students.

Finally, wishing to get things more into the open, I asked Dr. C. why he was using the term "growth" instead of "tumor" when talking with Mark. He replied that "growth" was a term that Mark himself had chosen to use. C. then said, "Mark has never asked me if it's cancer." I told him that Mark had made the statement "At least it's lymphatic, not cancerous." C. made no attempt to correct that deduction, but casually asked me if I knew what cancer was. I replied something about a destructive process that ate away at the body's cells, which, though quite incorrect, was what I thought cancer to be at that time. Incredibly, the subject was dropped, and I left the office with no greater understanding of the real nature of Mark's illness. Was that just denial on my part? Had the doctor been telling me and I refusing to hear and, like Mark, not asking the right questions?

I am astounded now at how misinformed I was then about tumors and cancer. Should my own ignorance have been reinforced by the doctor's silence? For whose sake was this silence being maintained—mine? Mark's? the surgeon's himself?

At least the exchange with C. that day brought about immediate results regarding Mark's diet. The head dietician made a personal visit to Mark's room that very afternoon to determine his favorite foods, and I was even allowed to bring in beer as another source of liquid protein. I was amazed at the clout of my personal request, and at the same time appalled to realize how necessary it had been for me to do anything at all. What if I'd never risked the asking?

When Dr. C. came the next day with the biopsy results, he did come in alone. He told us the "growth" had been formally diagnosed as "lymphosarcoma," but when Mark asked to have it spelled out so that I could write it down, C. said not to bother, that he'd do it for us later. He told us that Mark's case would now be turned over to the hematologist, a Dr. G., for treatment, and that while there was no longer any need for surgical procedure, he would have a continuing interest in Mark's case. It felt almost anticlimactic, after all my anticipated anxiety about the results, and while only slightly more informed, we were heartened by what appeared to be the doctor's casual tone.

I made no attempt to meet with Dr. C. out in the corridor, but when I saw him a short time later at the nursing station with his head resident surgeon, I did go up to them just to ask if there was anything else I should know. I was stunned to hear him reply, "Yes, the prognosis is not good." My immediate reaction was one of disbelief and anger that he should have kept such important information from *us* when I had especially asked that we be told the truth together.

I replied fiercely, "What? Tell me!" C. then said that Mark had two strikes against him—that because he was a young man, very rapid cell division was occurring in the abdominal cavity, and that the tumor had already reached an advanced stage. When I asked then, "How long are we talking about?" C. replied, "We're not talking in those terms." He assured me that there were many forms of treatment to try, various kinds of chemotherapy which gave at least short-range positive results, although the long-term effects were still unclear. When I said to him, "Why didn't you tell us, why didn't you tell Mark the truth?" he only replied, "Sometimes the truth can be very painful."

Although Mark knew nothing of my conversation with Dr. C. at the nurses' station, he was withdrawn and morose that evening. Little was said during visiting hours, and the strain of not sharing what more I now knew was deeply troubling to me, all the more so because we had trusted in the frankness of our session with the surgeon that afternoon. It was a difficult night at home for me. I knew my own energy and emotional levels were pretty low, and that I needed to tap new sources of strength for both of us.

Early the next morning, I placed a call to our friend Oliver Powell. No one answered, but I finally reached his wife Eleonore at her office.

I tried to explain what C. had said the day before, but started to cry instead. All I could manage to get out was "We need Oliver." Somehow, in spite of his being in conference until noontime, Eleonore got a message to him and he was on the first afternoon flight to us out of Boston. A friend offered to meet him at the airport (I still don't know how they made connections, as neither had seen the other before), and another friend offered to let him stay in her home. Although Mark slept through Oliver's first visit to the hospital, just having him with us was immediately comforting.

My father, too, was on his way, driving the eight hours alone to be with us.

It was the courageous caring of friends that initiated the next stage in our confrontation with the truth. Early the following morning, Mike Earnest's wife, Vicki, called and asked me to get in touch with Mike as soon as possible at the hospital. The Earnests were in our baby-sitting co-op and Robin often played with their little son. Mike was a resident in neurosurgery at the same hospital where Mark was now. While he had no direct connection with Mark's case, he knew the medical staff and was aware of the progress of Mark's illness.

Oliver and I went to the hospital together that day and found a friend from our Quaker Meeting already there. Russ had been talking with Mark, but when I came in he said, "I've really come to minister to Sandi today." Since he wished to talk with me alone, I left Oliver with Mark, and Russ and I went up to the hospital lounge.

Russ explained to me then that Gene, the young resident surgeon, was a neighbor of theirs, and that he had come to their home the previous evening. Gene knew of Russ's connection with us through Friends' Meeting, and so shared his concern that we were not being told the truth about Mark's condition. As chief resident under the operating surgeon, he was not free to reveal information to patients that had been withheld by his immediate superior, but he also knew of our concern for the truth and so told Russ some medical facts. Russ said to me now, "Lymphosarcoma, by medical definition, in any medical textbook, means cancer of the lymph. It is an extremely difficult form of cancer to treat, and perhaps it is time for you to begin dealing with that fact."

I learned later that others in my family had suspected cancer, and that the medical people around Mark, including Mike and Vicki, had known from the time of the surgery the nature of his illness. It was only now, however, that the term "cancer" had any reality for me in relation to Mark. My anger at not having been told the truth became an enabler for me. Directing the anger at the doctors, rather than at the disease, may have been my own "coping mechanism," for it gave me the strength to proceed with the information which Russ had offered.

I went to phone the hematologist now in charge of Mark's case. I made it clear that it was essential that I speak with him that very afternoon. I also called Mom Albertson and explained my wish to share the truth with Mark as soon as it had been verified by Dr. G. She felt strongly that Mark should not be told; she feared that knowing the diagnosis would only weaken him further and cause him to give up hope. Yet I knew him to be a strong person, and I believed in his ability to handle the truth about his own body.

Before I left the hospital at noontime, I went to find the resident in charge of Mark's ward that day and told him that Mark and I would probably be having a truth-telling session that afternoon. I asked that all medication be withheld that might cause Mark unclearness. The resident was amazingly receptive to my request and agreed to give only minimal medication for pain.

Oliver and my Dad went with me to Dr. G.'s office that afternoon, but I insisted on going in alone. While I have no real regrets about the way I proceeded, it would probably have been useful, as in any emotion-ally charged situation, to have another person present. Though I *feel* as if the conversation has been seared into my memory, it would have made sense to have a more objective person available to help verify what was in fact said. My own fiercely aroused sense of self and my anger from the morning made me feel I had to have this confrontation with the new doctor on my own. I wanted no more middlemen or intermediaries, even loving ones, "protecting" me or speaking for me.

I had met Dr. G. once before, but had never spoken alone with him. His office was very small, his desk covered with books and papers. I sat down and asked immediately, "Is lymphosarcoma a form of cancer?" When he answered yes, I said, "Then how long are we talking about for Mark?" He shuffled through some of the papers in front of him, picked out one, and read from a report that indicated an average life expectancy of five months. I felt, incredibly enough, a rush of relief. Mark was so very sick right then, I had feared we had no time left at all. Perhaps we would get to see this spring together after all; perhaps Mark would live to see the birth of our second child.

Dr. G. then went on to say that there was still a possibility that it was a form of Burkitt's tumor, a lymphatic growth with a history of successful X-ray therapy. G. still needed to examine the slides and lab results more closely, as Mark's symptoms were similar in many respects to those of a man now five years beyond diagnosis and still going strong. G. explained the various treatments possible, and the chemotherapy they would begin the next day.

I asked him to meet with Mark and me as soon as possible to share this information, but he replied, "Mrs. Albertson, some wives think their husbands should know the truth, but the patient may really not want to know it." I was dismayed by this put-down, and explained as clearly as I could that Mark and I had agreed prior to the surgery that we wanted to know the truth. Dr. G. told me to think about it overnight and then meet him outside Mark's room before his rounds the next morning.

I met Oliver and my Dad in the waiting room. I felt so relieved to have a hold on the truth, at least for myself, and so buoyed by the hope of five months and maybe even longer that my elation at reporting the average life expectancy with lymphosarcoma must have been rather startling. Oliver asked then if I was going to tell Mark what I had learned. When I said that I thought so, he replied, "Well, it's your covenant." If there had been any doubt in my mind as to how I would proceed, Oliver's words clarified and affirmed for me the ground upon which our relationship stood.

I had been wrestling with my reasons for telling Mark. Did I want to tell him the truth because I couldn't bear to carry it without him anymore? Yes, it was that in part. Aware of his strength, I needed to draw on it. I needed him to work out this problem with me, as we had worked out the various other dilemmas in our life together. Why should this, the most essential ultimate experience of the human condition, acknowledging the possibility of the death of someone you love, be done without that special person? If our past searchings and decisions had been based on respect for each other as individuals and on a commitment to stand in an open relationship with each other, then surely now, more than ever, that covenant needed to be honored. The withholding of the truth was keeping us from each other: it was wasting whatever time we had left to be together, to be really together. I left Oliver and my Dad and went into Mark's room.

CHAPTER
4
"Truth, Consequences, Promise . . ."

Mark was awake and more alert than he had been for some days. I got up on the bed, and holding his hands in mine, said, "Pooh, there's something we need to talk about." I told him that I'd just come from Dr. G.'s office, that I had learned for sure that the growth in his abdominal area was a tumor, and that lymphosarcoma was a form of cancer. I explained that it was a difficult one to control, but that there were many kinds of treatment to be tried and that we would do everything possible to fight it. I told him of the hope that it still might be a variation of Burkitt's tumor. I told him how the day had come about —about Russ and Gene's messages, of my anger at the surgeon, and of G.'s own reticence to share the truth with him.

His eyes filled with tears and he said, "And you had to carry this all alone." He declared that he was not "afraid" of the term "cancer," that he could handle that knowledge, and was proud that I had had the strength to go to the doctors and have it out with them.

We held each other then and cried together. The truth did set us free. I felt as if a huge weight had been lifted from me. What a relief to share it all at last, to end the constraint; to cry together, to laugh at our own pretendings, and give each other what we had to offer of strength and tenderness and caring. It was as if by acknowledging the enemy, we could now begin to come to terms with it, and do so together. As Pogo says, "We has met the enemy and they is us." Our covenant with each other was reaffirmed, and we could proceed with whatever living there was to be for us as a family.

While we lay talking together, a young man in medical attire came into the room. Though Mark recognized him, the man introduced himself to me as the anesthesiologist who had been present during

Mark's exploratory surgery. He asked if there was anything he could do for Mark, and explained that he would be on general duty that night. I was touched by his thoughtfulness and said that perhaps he could come by during the night to be with Mark.

It was interesting how we soon began to measure the people around us according to their ability and willingness to confront the truth with us—a kind of assessing of which doctors, which nurses or medical personnel were on our side; it was almost a game, a challenge to see who we could get to join us.

I left Mark after a bit and went to get Oliver so that he might have some time with Mark. Now that the seriousness of his condition was in the open, Oliver's visit made much more sense.

I found Oliver in the solarium. He had been weeping. He'd just talked long-distance with my twin Sue's husband David, and he spoke now of their need for each other as father and son. The possibility of the loss of someone special makes one more acutely aware of the fragility and finiteness of all loving relationships. Oliver said he had come to "minister" and found himself being ministered to as well. There was an odd juxtaposition of emotions at this particular point; Oliver was deeply saddened, while I felt strangely at peace, relieved—elated at knowing wholeness with Mark again.

Oliver went to Mark, and as I had hoped, the release from the pretense made possible an openness between them that would have been unlikely otherwise.

That evening was a good one for Mark and me. He spoke, incredibly enough, about remarriage for me, if or whenever he should die, and of the importance of not seeking someone like him, but of loving that person for himself, and of loving that person's children, if it should be so. We did, that night, for me at least, all the unfinished business we needed to do with each other, and I have never had a sense of things left unsaid.

It was long past visiting hours, but the nursing staff had not disturbed us. Most of the corridor lights had been turned off and the hospital was quiet. We held each other once more and exchanged the sign of peace —"Peace be unto thee." "And unto thee." Though not usually one to use ritualistic language, Mark gently added ". . . until death do us part."

I don't know how that night went for Mark. I don't know if the anesthesiologist ever stopped in, or whether Mark was awake if he did. I do know that part of my agonizing about telling Mark about his diagnosis had to do with the fact that he would be alone with that knowledge in his hospital bed that night. I was aware of how I would be held that night at home, with my parents and Mark's mother and Robin to surround and comfort me, and I ached for Mark, alone in that dimly lit, antiseptic setting. My mother rubbed my back and we had a cup of tea, a prelude to the many nights of sorrow and comforting that were to lie ahead.

I was already in Mark's room when Dr. G. came by on his rounds the next morning. He began, somewhat uncomfortably, by saying, "Mrs. Albertson has said she would like us to have a little talk." I told him then that Mark and I had already talked about his illness and that he was aware that he had a cancer of the lymph. Mark took over the conversation then and told G. that he did indeed want to know the truth. He went on to say, "If I have only three days left to live, I want to know it so I don't waste those three days." G. replied that he didn't play God like that, not anymore. He said that when he was younger, he used to give prognosis like "You have two years to live" or "three weeks to live," but that he'd been proved wrong too many times. Mark agreed that that was fair enough, but said, "Then just give us the medical facts, and we'll handle what that means for ourselves."

Dr. G. then explained the course of treatment that would begin that day. Since the tumor could not be removed surgically, chemotherapy would be used to arrest and counter its growth. They would be using Cytoxan initially to destroy the malignant cells. Cytoxan is a derivative of mustard gas, ironically a life-giving by-product of chemical warfare, recently released by the military for medical purposes. There were still many unknowns, since it was difficult to control the destruction of good cells as well. Yet it was a great relief to be embarked on a course of action at last.

It was a good session with G. What needed to be said about truth-sharing, about addressing Mark's illness honestly, had been said; the ground rules for our proceeding with each other, family and physician, had been laid, and Mark and I both had a good sense of being in Dr. G.'s care. Our trust in the medical world was reestablished, and we were not without hope.

CHAPTER
5
Time As a Gift

Remember all the things I once said I would do if I were going blind? Some of those ideas were really wild: go to Detroit to test-drive new turbo cars and fly to Hawaii to go surf-riding. But this is reality, buster! Come down to earth! Tuesday I won't be able to see a single thing.

There are hundreds of people who have been stricken with cancer and will die soon—not go blind—die! What do they do? Nothing —except keep on working as long as they can . . .

Before I fall asleep, I'll think of one thing to be thankful for—like tomorrow I *can* mow the lawn.

> —Excerpt from a high school composition
> "Only Three More Days to See"
> by Mark Albertson, age fifteen

Treatment began the afternoon of the day we talked with Dr. G. Mark's mother had returned to her home that morning, deeply troubled that nothing had yet been done to arrest or deter the course of the disease; she feared that the hospital was simply going to let Mark die. When she returned to visit twenty-four hours later, she was astounded. The effects of the Cytoxan were immediate and "miraculous." Within twelve hours, Mark's sweating stopped, his appetite improved, and the glazed look disappeared from his eyes. The tumor began to decrease in size, which meant that the tightness in his abdomen lessened and his breathing became easier. Sedation during the daytime was discontinued, and he became more lucid and more himself again.

Now began the long haul back to "recovery." Mark had lost twenty-five pounds in two weeks, and he was very weak. His liquid intake was of critical importance, as damage to the kidneys was a possible side-effect of the chemotherapy. Because there were still many unknowns about Cytoxan as a means of treatment, its beneficial effects needed to be constantly balanced against negative complications. We knew that this derivative of nitrogen mustard was killing off the cancerous cells; what else it might be destroying was not always clear.

The phone rang at home during breakfast a few mornings later, and it took me a moment to realize that it was Mark's voice on the other end, asking if I would bring some pajamas into the hospital for him that day. He was finally rebelling against the hospital "johnny." That he was well enough to perform even this simple act of calling home was a victory.

As Mark continued to improve, he began to long for those areas of personal control which one takes for granted when in good health. Simple things like being able to take a bath or wash his hair were still determined and scheduled by others. When an aide was unavailable, his mother asked to be allowed to help, so that Mark could take a tub bath, his first since the hospitalization began. What a simple pleasure, so easily taken for granted.

We were all overjoyed by Mark's "return to life." It was proof to me that the treatment was working, that we were winning. I had no knowledge of the course that a cancer takes. I had never heard of the term "remission"; I did not know that Mark was in one, that remissions were typical, yet often only an interruption, a temporary respite from the onward course of the disease. Mark's rapid recovery, for us a cause for rejoicing, in fact only confirmed the doctors' worst fears about the nature and outcome of this perverse disease. Perhaps it is just as well that we did not know the whole story, at least not then. As it was, nothing now dampened the enthusiasm with which we proceeded with life.

On January 19, seven days after the beginning of treatment, and twenty-three days after he'd first been admitted, Mark was released from the hospital. Before we left, I took down the photographs, mobiles and drawings by Robin that I had used to cover the barren walls, and put in their place a large sign that read: MARK ALBERTSON HAS GONE HOME. We joined the flow of people along the outpatient corridor. Mark was in the world again, and we kept looking at each other and grinning.

Outside the hospital entrance, a few forsythia blossoms still clung to the bush that we had seen more than three weeks before. Perhaps we would see spring together again after all.

Mom Albertson drove us home, as I was now too pregnant for the driver's seat, and then she went on to her own house. Robin was waiting at our doorway, and she hurled herself into Mark's arms from the porch steps. My sister, Sue, had arrived from Chicago to help us out and share our joy.

I had assumed that the afternoon would be spent resting, but Mark wanted very much to get outdoors again. At his suggestion, we piled into the car, dog and all, and Sue drove us to a large park on the outskirts of the city. Although it was still only mid-January, it was a delightfully mild springlike day, and we ambled along the wooded paths, a family again.

We prepared a salubrious, budget-bending dinner for that evening and broke open a special bottle of wine. That night our typically silent Quaker grace was punctuated with a rousing chorus of "Hallelu."

Mark seemed to be on the mend. His appetite was voracious and I often woke to hear him rattling around in the kitchen. I would get up then and join him for a fried-egg sandwich. It was good to lie with him and be held by him again, to have back rubs and wing-tucks at the end of the day and to fall asleep in the curve of his body. We moved in a kind of euphoria now, marked by an unarticulated yet poignant sense of the preciousness of our time together.

Mark could not remember Oliver's visit at all. When I reminded him of the time they had spent on that truth-telling day, he began to weep. It was distressing to him to have lost touch with reality in that way, and he was appalled at his confusion and loss of memory; he thought the conversation he'd had with Oliver had been only a dream. When he learned that Oliver had purchased the stereo system which he had recommended that day, Mark was amused and reassured that at least his judgment at that time had been trustworthy.

We decided to have friends in again, eating simple meals together as we had before Mark's illness. Though we weren't sure if it was an appropriate thing to do, we called Gene, the young resident surgeon, to ask if he and his wife, Maryanna, could join us. Maryanna had a meeting scheduled for the evening we were suggesting, so we promised them a rain check for another time. A few minutes later Gene called back to ask if he could come anyway, without his wife. He was aware, as we were not, of how suspect was our ability to honor such a rain check. We were touched by his response, by his willingness to meet us outside the professional medical setting, and we finally changed the date of the dinner so that everyone could come. When Gene asked Mark how he was feeling, Mark laughed and said, "Well, *you* might take it with a grain of salt, but I feel great." That evening meant the nurturing of old and new friendships and the breaking of bread. It ended with all of us in the kitchen washing the dishes.

By the first of February, ten days after his release from the hospital, Mark was back at school full-time, working on his master's thesis and teaching classes. He was determined to make up for lost time, since graduation was to be the third week in May. Once again he was at his desk late into the night.

Mark took the Cytoxan medication in pill form at home now, along with prednisone and Allopurinol. For someone who used to refuse even an aspirin, it was hard to be so dependent on pills. It became clear that the medication would have to be continued for some time, indefinitely perhaps, as a protective measure. So far there'd been no negative side-effects (other than the need to drink a lot of fluids), and if pills meant ensuring a longer life, then he conceded it was worth the hassle. He attended to his own medications and got on with his work.

Mark had outpatient status, and went in every week or two for a checkup. Dr. G. knew we were on a tight budget. He told us that we would not receive a bill from him, so I sent him loaves of home-made bread ("bushels of wheat" currency) whenever Mark had an appointment. Mark drove to school instead of bicycling as he had in the past, but his strength was returning rapidly. He gained back twelve pounds, though he was disgusted that it was mostly fat and not muscle. He made arrangements to swim in the university pool, and asked his mother to bring along his old ice skates from college days on her next visit.

Mark's mother came to stay for a few days early in February. The evening she arrived Mark told her what he wished to have happen to his body when he died. The two of us had already talked it over, but

I especially wanted his mother to know Mark's wishes directly from him, preferably at a time of ease among us all. He was quite clear about wanting his body given to medical research and said that he did not wish to take up earth and space that should be left for the living. (In his studies of urban mass transportation, he'd always been outraged at instances of families being evicted from their homes because of highway development while those same routes were diverted around cemeteries.) He asked that at some time after his death there be a memorial service at a Quaker meeting house, but told his mother that if she wished some kind of service within their family's tradition—United Church of Christ —as well, that would be fine. Although he hoped that we would be able to carry out his wishes, he knew that both his mother and I were troubled by the fact that donation to medical research meant cremation and burial by the medical institution rather than the family. (That state law has since been changed to allow for family disposal of the cremated remains.) He finally said, "What happens afterward is really for your sakes, so do what you need to do." His gift to us was to let us know his wishes, and then to free us to proceed as we were able.

We wrote a letter to friends and family which we planned to send along with the birth announcement of our soon-to-arrive second child. The letter spoke openly of the nature of Mark's illness, yet optimistically of the treatment. Things were going so well now that the statistic of a five-month life expectancy seemed almost too melodramatic to mention. We did include it in the letter finally. Even though we didn't talk about it much, I think we both knew, deep down, that we weren't really in the clear yet, that we were still in a "meanwhile," and we decided not to pretend with friends about the future.

February 1972

Dear Friends and Relations,

Three days after Christmas, we rushed back to Philadelphia to admit Mark to the hospital. After nine days of tests, exploratory surgery was performed, and we learned that he has lymphosarcoma, a malignant tumor of the lymph system in the abdominal cavity. It could not be removed surgically, and the prognosis was not good. The tumor was already quite large and composed of rapidly dividing cells. Statistics suggested an average life expectancy of five months. Several kinds of medical treatment remain available, however, and chemotherapy has begun. Mark's response to the Cytoxan has been very positive and we are much encouraged . . . While this continues, Mark is able to be treated as an outpatient, and he's feeling so good, he has resumed work at school on his teaching assistantship and thesis research.

These have been full and challenging days for us. We went through a truth-telling crisis with the doctors who felt that patients should not be told they have cancer. Finally, against their counsel, but with a deep sense that our covenant of honesty with each other was of primal importance, San told Mark everything about his condition. Our covenant was renewed, and we were freed to go on through the medical facts to deal with the human emotional aspects of a quite possibly terminal disease. Together we have been seeking a balance between realistic hope and preparedness. We are thankful for whatever time there is to share together this tragic and joyful sense of life.

There has been, throughout it all, a prevailing sense of being upheld—of strength drawn from beyond oneself—most often in the form of the loving, deeply caring support of family and friends: the long bus and car trips alone by parents; Oliver's much needed presence on two hours' notice; Sue's week here from Chicago to share deep tears and laughter; spring bouquets in the midst of a winter storm, one for Mark at the hospital and one for me at home; homemade bread, taxi service and Robin-care; written and spoken messages of support, and quiet presences; and all those offers made though perhaps not realized.

The concern and support have come both from old and previously untapped sources, and the by-products of Mark's illness have been immeasurable. A Quaker Meeting that had spent much of its energy in busyness and committees has become a genuinely caring community, actualizing its capacity for love with a new sense of what it means to be "Christs to one another." Friends with whom we had previously shared only paper-bag lunches or fondue and child care have given of time and energy and quiet caring. Young doctors struggling with the truth issue in terminal cases became involved in our truth-sharing process. Friends who have been out of touch for several years have reached across time and distance to give support. The whole process of persons meeting persons, strength meeting strength, of being ministered to and ministering unto, has been a cyclical one.

There has been, especially, a renewed sense that there does exist, at the depth of all of our beings, a creating, loving, sustaining force, linking us to one another, to which we are ultimately bound and by which we are upheld.

And so, we go about the business of living, with joy for whatever this meanwhile holds—each day of being a family together, a special bonus.

"Hope is the thing with feathers that perches in the soul."

—Emily Dickinson

Love,
San and Mark and
Robin

There were a few friends with whom we had been close in the past who did not respond to this February letter. Their inability or unwillingness to share this dimension of our experience meant a barren space between us, and because of it, these relationships have had their own closure or little death.

The relationships that did grow and deepen were with those friends who risked confronting the truth with us. We rarely talked about death itself, yet there was an unspoken acknowledgment that we could not all assume the future with each other, and our times together became the more treasured.

In early February my obstetrician announced that the baby might arrive anytime. Though I had had to have a Caesarean delivery for our first child, Dr. A. now commented during one office visit that if I should go into labor before the date planned for the surgery, perhaps I could deliver the child normally. I said nothing at the time, yet I was dismayed and frightened at the possibility of going into labor with no updating of the Lamaze training we had started earlier. I had no desire to take any risks for myself or the baby, and I became increasingly fearful.

At last I told Mark how troubled I was. He leaned across the breakfast table, picked up the phone, called the doctor and explained that we needed to be assured that no unnecessary risk would be taken, and the ambiguity about procedure was cleared up between us all. I was immeasurably grateful to Mark. It was a comfort now to have someone else in charge for a change, to have Mark be the strong one again.

Mark had asked the obstetrician if he could be present during our child's birth, and even though it was to be a surgical delivery, the doctor had agreed. He had told Mark to scrub up on the day of the delivery and to wait until he was signaled to enter the operating room. I was fully conscious that morning, having chosen to be under only local anesthesia. While the anesthesia was taking effect, the head nurse appeared at my side and announced that due to hospital regulations, my husband could not be present. I was in no position to argue. Dr. A. arrived shortly thereafter, however, and declared that hospital regulations notwithstanding, Mark would be allowed in as soon as the baby was ready to leave the uterus. Dr. A. knew then, as we did not, how very little time we probably had left together as a family. (The whole timing of this pregnancy and birth was to seem providential in retrospect. I'd become pregnant as soon as Mark and I had decided to try to have another child. Then, in the second month, I was exposed to German measles, and an anxious time had ensued; we wondered whether the pregnancy ought to be terminated. All seemed well, however, so we decided to go ahead with it.)

Now Mark came to stand beside me, and it wasn't long before a strange gurgling sound could be heard. Although still in the embryonic sac, this little one was proclaiming her eagerness to be out in the world. Radiant, Mark announced that Kimberly had arrived. As one friend has said, "The only thing nicer than one little girl is two little girls." Mark stayed with Kim while she was bathed and weighed in another section of the operating room.

A few days later, we all celebrated Robin's third birthday in the lounge outside the maternity ward. We tried to make a merry party, but Robin had a bad cold, and Mark, a painful ear infection—his first since childhood, caused now by the chemotherapy's breakdown of the body's resistance to ordinary germs. Though Mark had been coming in as often as possible to visit, I insisted now that he stay home and get rested.

I was in the hospital for ten days following surgery. One of my roommates was a young teenager on methadone, whose prematurely born child was going through heroin withdrawal. Another, a Hispanic, had just delivered her third child, and was struggling with the doctor's advice to have her tubes tied, a move she favored but her husband opposed. It was a heady setting for reflections on the quality of life. With a newborn child I was more aware than ever these days of endings and beginnings, and all the life held in between.

Although we knew we'd need some extra help at home for a while following my surgery, Mark laid aside his research so the four of us could have a few days alone when Kim and I first came home. It began snowing lightly that first evening out of the hospital, and when a young friend from our Meeting stopped by, we left him with the sleeping children for a little while, and went for a walk around our neighborhood. It was one of those quiet magical nights, with new snow covering the grunge of the city; the air, clear and still. We walked gently through the snow, speaking of the new life in our family.

The next evening we had a love feast, a special meal for just the two of us. We prepared some favorite recipes together—broiled shrimp, green beans supreme, riced potatoes—and used the good china with candlelight and wine. I scheduled Kim's nursing so that both children would be fed and tucked into bed early, and then changed into a favorite nonmaternity dress that had been in the closet for months. Just as we sat down for the first course, onion soup, Kimberly started crying. I could have wept, I was so tired of being on call. I shut all the doors between us and her cradle, but at last Mark went and got her. He perched her in a little recliner beside him, where she lay for the rest of the meal, content to watch the candlelight.

Mark spent much of the day now at the university. His thesis in rough draft was due the first of April and he was really pushing. One evening I went out after the children were in bed, leaving him to work on the thesis. He was changing Kim's diapers when I returned, and admitted that he had spent most of the evening holding and rocking her.

Although the doctor said he was doing fine, Mark wasn't so sure. His stomach felt full all the time and he was very tired. I only saw improvement, yet our friends noticed how gaunt and aged he looked. My college roommate, who'd come from out of state to help after she received our letter, later told me that she'd had a sense of last things when she said goodbye to Mark at the train station. The conductor had been impatient and sarcastic, and when he railed at her for what seemed to be an improper ticket, she'd wanted to scream at him, "Don't you know my friend is dying!" Perhaps the conductor was carrying a burden of his own that day; how little we know about the lives and pain of others.

The emotional and physical strain of the past two months began to tell on both of us. Mark finally called his mother to ask if she could come to be with us again for a few days. The morning after she arrived, Mark seemed to take forever to get going; he hung around the house, complaining that he wasn't feeling so good. I was quite put out with him —the apartment always seemed so much smaller when someone lived in with us—and asked crossly if he shouldn't get to the office and get some work done. He finally left for school, and I went about the business of wringing out diapers.

Just before lunch, the phone rang. It was Mark. He'd stopped off at the student health clinic, and said now, as if he'd been commenting on the weather, "The tumor's growing back again. Dr. G. wants me in the hospital this afternoon." Our victory over this disease—all that we had begun to assume again about our right to a normal family life—came to an abrupt halt. The remission was over.

Mark drove home and once again we packed a small suitcase. He stuffed his thesis materials into his battered old briefcase, determined not to be thwarted in his attempt to get it done for graduation, and the two of us drove back to the university medical center. Thus began round two. Dr. G. was really provoked with Mark for not coming to him directly when he hadn't been feeling well, for having "dropped into" the student health clinic. We had been trying so hard not to overreact or become paranoid about physical ailments—how were we to know that fatigue or constipation or general malaise were some kind of warning sign?

Though we were caught off-guard by the return of the tumor, it came as no surprise to the medical people around us. Any cells that would respond to the Cytoxan by disappearing so easily would be capable of returning as quickly. If Mark had recovered more slowly initially, or if he had been an older man, his chances of recovery would have been far better. The irony was that as a young man in his prime, however, he had a very healthy tumor. The oral form of Cytoxan medication that Mark had been taking at home had failed to arrest the growth of the cancerous cells. Mark had come to the end of the first "stay of execution." This disease had its own agenda, and the fight for more time began anew. Health was to become the interlude, with the natural course of the disease the main acts of the drama. What one tries to direct is a play with longer "intermissions" in a tragedy that has little to offer for comic relief.

That evening, when I went to Mark's room at visiting time, I apologized for having been so bitchy that morning, for not realizing or being willing to acknowledge that he might really be sick again. I climbed into bed with him (no mean thing in a hospital setting where one of the greatest losses is that of privacy, and one anticipates being thrown out for putting one's hand under the covers). That time together helped to heal the rough edges that had grown between us. We could no longer assume that life together was some inviolable right; we knew we needed to keep our love for each other up to date.

Mark continued to work on his thesis as much as possible, though hospital schedule and environment are not very conducive to concentration or creativity. He also wanted to get back into shape physically. Determined to build up his backpacking and child-carrying muscles for the summer, he asked to be allowed to work out in the physical-therapy unit. He returned from his first visit to the P.T. clinic greatly sobered by the condition of those he saw around him. The sight of one young man in a wheelchair struggling to lift a spoon to his mouth stunned him, and he said he would never again assume the body's capacity to perform such tasks. In the lounge we overheard a young man say to an older couple about his wife, "Well, we'll know in a few hours whether it's malignant." It was startling; our preoccupation with ourselves was tempered by this awareness of the suffering of others.

The tumor took longer to abate this time, and fluid in Mark's abdominal cavity caused difficulty in his breathing again. Mark wished to know as much as possible about what was happening to him, and a friend of ours who is a nurse gave us a long medical description of Cytoxan, its effects and side-effects. There was no staff pretense during this hospital stay. Mark openly asked questions and demanded answers. He discussed sections from Dr. Elisabeth Kübler-Ross's book *On Death and Dying* with some of the young resident doctors.

The most important "outside" help for me during this whole time was a Pendle Hill Quaker publication, *Dear Gift of Life*, sent to us by a Friend from our old Meeting in Cambridge. A collection of thoughts and writings by Bradford Smith as he faced his own death by cancer, it is a beautiful and moving acknowledgment of the creative role which death plays in the ongoingness of life.

A special pattern of communication developed between Robin and Mark during this hospitalization. Each morning Mark phoned home to tell her about the animal picture on the sugar packet that he had saved from his breakfast tray. One morning Robin explained to Mark that she had a cold, and then, with three-year-old directness, asked, "What do you have, Daddy?" After a pause he replied, "I have cancer." She handed the phone to me and said, "I think Daddy's crying." Though he had never hesitated to discuss his illness with others who asked, he was deeply shaken by the weight of Robin's question and the implications of his answer.

Robin and I sneaked in visits a number of times during this hospitalization, meeting Mark upstairs in the solarium. Once, as the visiting period came to an end, she began to sob that she didn't want to leave her daddy. Mark had to get off the elevator at his floor, and we went on down to the lobby. Robin continued to sob as we headed toward the parking lot. It had begun to rain, but I stopped in the middle of the sidewalk and tried to comfort her, explaining that we would be back again. Suddenly her tears came to an abrupt halt. With the resiliency of a child, she lifted her head and announced in disgust, "The rain is splashing my stockings!"

My schedule was crazy those days. I tried to be with Mark at least once or twice a day, continuing to nurse Kim between hospital visits. I recovered rapidly from my own surgery because I had to. It's hard, at such a time, to keep track of priorities, and it was hard, I'm sure, on those who helped take care of Kim that I chose to nurse her. There were many times when I came dashing into the house from the hospital to a little one who had chosen a different feeding schedule that evening. I always left bottles of sugar water or prepared formula for just such times, but Kim was not easily diverted. Though it wasn't easy to be the relaxed

nursing mother pictured by the La Leche League, it was such a comfort
to me to care for Kim in this way that I wished to continue it as long
as possible. It was my own selfish need to have that closeness to our
newborn, to maintain, in the midst of all the helpers that surrounded
us, a special relationship with her that couldn't be satisfied by anyone
else.

In times of family crisis, it's hard for everyone involved to be clear
about where one's time and energies are needed most. Mark was glad
for whatever time I could spend with him, sometimes forgetting, in that
unnatural world of the hospitalized, all the other demands that were
placed on me as well. It seemed to me at the time that the children were
doing fine; there were many loving people around to care for them. My
mother told me, though, that there were nights when she tucked a
sobbing Robin into bed.

There were many friends who offered to care for Robin and Kim
during Mark's hospitalizations, but we turned more often to our own
families in order to maintain as stable and familiar a setting for the
children as possible. It did help, nonetheless, when our friends included
the children in their activities. A friend came one day just to spend some
time with Robin, talking on the front porch and playing with some toys
her own children had sent along. Others took Robin on outings to a
neighborhood puppet show or school play. A young father from our
Meeting invited Robin to join his kids on several afternoons when he
was responsible for their care.

Late one afternoon a woman from another Friends' meeting in the
city arrived on our doorstep, bearing a complete dinner for our family.
I'd never met her, but she explained that she'd heard of us through other
Quakers. I had little energy, just then, for building any new relationships, and I was grateful for the comfortableness with which this "stranger" offered comfort without requiring active response or involvement
from me.

Another evening, just as Robin and I had finished supper, the doorbell
rang. It was a young mother in our babysitting co-op whom I knew only
slightly. She said, "I've come to do your dishes," and she did. Though
it felt a bit awkward at first, it gets me grinning whenever I think of it
now. There is a new level of trusting reached when you can allow a friend
to know your "encrustations"—to vacuum your house or clean the
bathroom.

There are difficulties, however, in being so dependent on the help of others. It was exhausting to have others living with us, especially in our small quarters, and no easy matter to negotiate the housing arrangements when more than two parents were there at the same time. The anxiety of those around me, especially when Mark was in the hospital, often served to drive my own anxiety deeper; I found myself keeping up a cheerful exterior to counterbalance the despair of others. Trying to maintain outward peace in our household, I was left little space for expressing my own feelings.

This strangled emotion often had a way of being laid on Robin. Confused and troubled herself by her father's absence, she would often find herself being reprimanded by more than one adult for the same thing or held accountable to differing standards of discipline. Crises bring out the best and the worst in us, and it would be wrong to expect that there would be no dark places, even in the most loving and supportive of families. It was often Mark, with his perspective and humor, who played the role of conciliator from his hospital bed.

One gift our friends gave was to help me to remember that I was still a person myself, that life still needed to proceed for me. They sensed how much I needed relief, even if briefly, from both the house and hospital routine. I needed music and art and exposure to creative, nonmedical things. One friend gave us passes to the zoo; another took Robin and me to a flower show in the city. Mom Albertson, when she was with us, also needed outlets and diversions, and though they did not know her well at the time, two older friends of mine asked her to join them for a tour of the city's historical homes. Such activities initiated by our friends did much to relieve the tension in this period; they provided a constructive chance for all of us to get distance from each other for a while so that we could come back more relaxed and whole.

As soon as he was strong enough, Mark was granted a few hours' pass from the hospital. I brought in street clothes for him (how he delighted in the smell of his old leather boots!) and the two of us went to an exhibition by local artists, a block from the hospital. Mark needed to rest a lot, but he wandered slowly among the paintings, savoring this freedom.

On another pass we went as a family to a forest area on the outskirts of the city. When I told Robin that we were going to the hospital to bring her dad home for an outing, her face turned radiant and she exclaimed, *"My* daddy? *My* daddy's coming *home?"* I could hardly bear to tell her it was just for a few hours. She sat next to him in the middle seat of our microbus while I drove, her eyes on Mark throughout the trip. It was a delightfully mild March day, and Robin and our dog, Manda, raced around us through the woods. I took photographs of Robin flinging herself into Mark's arms and of the two of them bending over some discovery in the spring earth. When it was time to leave Mark off at the hospital, Robin refused to give him a kiss or say goodbye, her abrupt withdrawal revealing how hard these separations were on her.

Mark was in the hospital for twelve days until his condition stabilized sufficiently for him to be considered "in remission" once more. Though he needed to continue to receive the Cytoxan intravenously, Dr. G. agreed to give it to him in his office, so that Mark did not have to remain hospitalized. As the two of us rode down in the elevator the day of his release, I pounded on the elevator wall with my fists, shouting, "We're leaving for good this time, and we're never coming back." We walked to the Student Union for some hot chocolate together. Then Mark went over to his office to do some work on his thesis, and I drove home.

To have had the first remission last so briefly was a sobering lesson. Mark continued to explore job possibilities for the following fall. Though we talked of camping plans with friends for the summer and a trip to Chicago after graduation to see Sue and Dave, it was a time for reexamining priorities. My parents offered to care for the children if Mark and I wished to take a trip. I would have loved for all of us to go on a camping trip then, but it was still only March and we would have had to go some distance to be warm enough. Mark was clear about wanting to finish his thesis and I really wanted to keep nursing Kim a while longer. So given the nature of our hope then, we decided to proceed as normally as possible. One morning at breakfast I said, "Even if something should happen to you, I don't think I'd want to have spent this time any differently," and Mark agreed.

Around this time we all had bad colds, and I was becoming increasingly exhausted and worried about Kim, whose congestion caused her trouble breathing. It was hard to admit that we needed still more help from others. It was hard not to be in control, not to be able to carry out the roles of parent/provider/graduate student as competently and self-sufficiently as we had envisioned ourselves doing. Yet one morning we all reached our limit, and in desperation I phoned my oldest sister, Cil, in Vermont, to ask if there was any chance she could come be with us. It meant leaving her own family of four and her teaching job, yet she said she would be there the next day. When Mark had first become sick, Cil had alerted her department chairman that she might need to take some personal leave days. She had been waiting ever since, while my folks and my other sister had come, waiting for a chance to help. I was to learn a lot during Mark's illness about the cycle of giving and receiving.

A few days after Cil arrived, Mark discovered a lump on his neck. It looked as if the tumor might be spreading to other lymph areas. We left Cil with the children and went together to the hospital student clinic.

It was Saturday afternoon, with few staff members on duty. There'd been a serious ice hockey injury and we waited over an hour before a doctor was available. Two young coeds sat opposite us in the waiting room, comparing their latest symptoms. "My throat is killing me." "I had such a headache, I thought I'd die." I wanted to shake them and tell them to stop their sniveling; it was hard not to be self-righteous about our own crisis.

When the clinic doctor finally examined Mark, he explained that the lumps were simply caused by steroids, often a side-effect of the medication. It would have been nice to have known ahead of time; it certainly would have saved us a long Saturday afternoon in the waiting room. The anxiety of discovery and self-analysis by a patient may be far worse than the foreknowledge of possible complications or side-effects. We were told by the clinic doctor, then, that the steroids might even produce the effect of hunchbackness—no small matter, but at least knowing gave us time to digest that possibility and joke about it.

I felt both immensely relieved and at the same time almost let down by the simple explanation of the lumps. Keeping a balanced perspective on this whole disease process was not easy. It is easier to ask for help when things are really bad, and it was almost as if this alarm, this trip to the hospital—had it signaled a serious change—would have justified Cil's visit.

Cil and I and the children went to our Friends' Meeting for Worship the next Sunday morning. Meeting had always been an important clarifying, renewing time in the week for me. I needed the silence and the "centering down" which is the focus of our Quaker worship, and I needed the nonverbal as well as the verbal expressions of support which this community provided.

I never asked, "Why us? Why is this happening to our family?" We might as easily have said, "Why not us?" I do not worship a God who actively wills disaster for individuals or families. Miracles, for me, take the form of an intricate spiderweb or the birth of a child. Bradford Smith's pamphlet spoke clearly to our own thoughts about what was happening: "Disease and accident happen without regard to moral worth. The why of natural law is in its way as beautiful as a work of art. We need not blame God for viruses and cancer and car accidents. God is spirit, the embodiment of all that a good man knows how to conceive and more."[1] Like Smith, we accepted our place within the laws of nature and willingly took "our chances in that vast splendid creation." Having addressed the possibility of death, we turned from it to go about the business of living. The human mind cannot usually retain for long the concept of death: we simply did not believe the prognosis of five months —not yet.

CHAPTER
6
Closures

It is typical of any grave illness that one ricochets back and forth between crisis and relief, dismay and hope. Although the lumps on Mark's neck turned out to be insignificant, he told us when we returned from Meeting that Sunday morning that he could feel the tumor again through the abdominal wall.

A friend called a few hours later to say that he'd reserved seats for us at the Academy of Music performance that evening. We decided to go; time left for just the two of us felt more fragile now than ever.

When we arrived at the Academy, we discovered that the seats reserved for us were not together—the tickets themselves, a symbol of our own reality. Mark sat several rows in front of me, and I watched him, through the theater darkness, acutely aware of the distance between us, conscious that this might be our last chance at such an event. We met during intermission and finally found two empty seats together. The second half of the program was a performance of Respighi's *Pines of Rome*. We'd been in Rome together five years before, on our way home from the Peace Corps, and were swept up now by the music's images —children playing by the pines at the Villa Borghese, the nightingale's full-throated moonlit song, and the vision of Rome's grandeur at dawn. We bought an album of the music a few days later, knowing that it marked a special space in our time together, then and now.

Oliver and Eleonore's daughter, Loey, came to spend her Easter college break with us. She found Mark considerably changed physically, his features puffy from the medication and his whole body weakened by the tumor. She's said since that she had wanted to sit down and cry with us, but that it never really seemed appropriate to do so. Mark did take her hand at one point, and laying it on his abdomen said, "Here's where the cancer is." She understood him to mean "Take me seriously. This is my reality." Yet Mark's illness was not generally a topic of conversation. It wasn't that we were trying to avoid the issue; we simply preferred to dwell in the present, rather than in the unknown future.

On Easter Saturday we all went for a walk, children and dog included, in a wooded section outside the city. It was an early April morning, Kim's first expedition to the woods—and Mark's last. Mark was wearing his favorite old climbing boots and woodsman's jacket, but his face was drawn and strained, his eyes, deep-sunk and darkly circled. He carried Kim on his back at first, but soon asked me to take over.

Loey shot a roll of film that morning. She was a good unobtrusive photographer, and conscious of the weight of those scenes. The air was full of spring sounds and smells, and there was a bittersweet wondering for us about our place amidst all this life.

Though we'd walked less than an hour, Mark asked me to drive home. There we found an Easter lily at the door, left by a young friend from New England who'd been on a wilderness camping trip that Mark and I had helped chaperon for a high school group. Though we hadn't seen Jay for two years, we had written him of Mark's illness in February. A note said, "Sorry to have missed you. Will try to see you soon." We would have stayed home that morning had we known Jay was coming, and we felt disappointed and frustrated.

Easter Sunday, about twenty people came to our house for breakfast. We've always loved having friends in for breakfast, especially Easter morning, and it seemed right to have our Meeting join us in our own home this year as well. Everyone brought something to help and we spread out on the living room floor to paint Easter eggs. Some who came were startled by Mark's physical appearance, for he had lost more hair and was considerably thinner. Loey observed that while some people seemed unsure of what to say or do initially, neither Mark nor I seemed troubled or uncomfortable in that gathering, which diffused the awkwardness.

Meeting for Worship was held at another home later that morning. Our group was small and often totally silent for the duration of the hour of worship. Yet after I left the Meeting room that morning to put Kim down to sleep, it was Mark who offered the first message. He'd spoken only once before in Meeting. Now he spoke about his illness and the quality of life. Loey, who'd been on the verge of tears the whole morning, was startled to hear Mark speak of Jesus—not usually a part of his vocabulary—and of the model for living he offered. Mark made some reference to learning from Jesus how to die as well, but the emphasis was on the Galilean's life rather than on his death. Mark made no bid for sympathy and did no egotistical posturing.

A few moments later another young man, a visitor who did not know Mark, made a disparaging remark about Biblical references and spoke at length about the value of natural foods and astrological signs over medical science. His put-down of Mark's message broke the spirit of the Meeting, and the silence, usually centered and calming, felt uncomfortable and strained that morning. Meeting ended for me with a sense of frustration at the limits of our human ministry to each other. We shared the usual tea and coffee cake, and then we went off to hide Easter eggs and fly kites on a nearby hillside.

The next day Mark went in for a checkup at Dr. G.'s office. He was doing the routine breathing exercise, saying, "Ninety-nine, ninety-nine," while the doctor thumped his back, when Dr. G. suddenly said, "Shit!" He'd detected the presence of fluid, a sign that the tumor was back at work. Dr. G. made some gruff apology for his language, but Mark replied wryly, "I'm glad to know you care."

Dr. G. decided to use radiation to counter the tumor and Mark entered the hospital for the third time that afternoon, located this time in a wing particularly designated for severe arthritic, heart and cancer patients. It was an older section of the hospital and much more humane. The tone was less blatantly efficient and professional; the atmosphere, less antiseptic. There was more familiarity between the patients and staff.

A young clinical nursing instructor had heard earlier about Mark from some of the residents in the hospital. Phyllis had returned to nursing instruction following the difficult hospitalization and death of a close friend. Her central concern now was the sensitizing of young students to the care of persons with a terminal illness. She and Mark talked about children (hers and ours) and the process of his illness. She was also a Quaker, and as it turned out, lived only a few blocks away from us.

When Phyllis stopped in to see him the next day, Mark was on the phone with Robin, and when he hung up, he began to weep. She held him in her arms, silently sharing his tears.

Robin was able to visit her father once during this hospitalization. I'd made new spring dresses for the two of us, bright flowered prints, in intentionally lively colors, and we wore them that day for the first time. We met in an alcove along the hallway of the main downstairs lobby. It was strange to sit on a small stiffly upholstered couch, Robin and I in our spring dresses, Mark in his pajamas, as people bustled back and forth along the corridor only an arm's-length away. Robin and Mark read and drew pictures together, but he spoke little. He told me later that it had been a hard visit for him, that he'd felt about to burst with his own aching for a normal life with us.

I came upon him the next day at his hospital window, watching the cherry trees in bloom and the students on their way to classes. He spoke with sadness and some bitterness about those who chose to smoke or use drugs, consciously participating in a process that could be destructive to their own systems. His own body, well and whole, would be a high enough for him.

Early one morning, a few days after the X-ray therapy had begun, Mark called and asked if I could come be with him for a little while. His mother was there to stay with the children, so I dressed and went right in to the hospital. He had weighed himself already that morning, just before he called, and when he saw that there had been no significant weight change, it confirmed his fear that the tumor and the fluid were not receding this time. He was weeping when I entered the room and we held each other for a while. It was the first time since we'd known of the diagnosis that I'd seen him with so little hope. He said to me then, "It's not that I'm afraid of dying; I just don't want to give up so much life."

We decided to ask Dr. G. for another assessment of where we were medically, and I stayed with Mark until the doctor came in on his morning rounds. Mark asked him whether it was realistic anymore for him to put energy into job applications for the fall. Dr. G. was unusually brusque, and made some comment about it being presumptuous for anyone to plan too far ahead. He told Mark that he would not have a normal life expectancy, and said, when we asked about the treatments, "After everything has been done that we can do, you will probably have no longer than a month." Mark made it clear to Dr. G. that morning that he did not wish to be kept alive by extraordinary measures. I asked if it would be possible for Mark to be at home "at the end," perhaps even at his mother's home in the country where he'd grown up and where he could hear birds sing again. Dr. G. replied, "Whatever you wish." We'd covered some pretty heavy territory in that brief exchange.

April tenth arrived, the day the first draft of Mark's thesis was due. Mark called the head of his department from the hospital room to say that the draft was not ready and that graduation was no longer his major goal. He explained that he was rearranging priorities for his life now and wished to spend as much time as possible with his family. Dr. Carr understood; he'd been amazed, in fact, that Mark had kept at his work as long as he had.

On April eleventh, Mark was released from the hospital. Although the radiation treatment had made him quite weak, he asked if we could ride out to the countryside for a little while. On the way home we had engine trouble, and Mark went to work under the hood. Whatever it was that he did worked, and we made it home, grateful for the special skills which he still brought to our lives.

His abdomen had decreased only slightly during this last hospitalization, and now became noticeably more swollen as the days went on. The X-ray treatments continued; Mark went in for them on an outpatient basis each morning on his way to the university. He chose to keep working on his thesis, though the pressure to meet academic deadlines was off. When he spoke of the future, Mark said that all he wanted now vocationally was a nine to five job so that he could spend more time at home. He stopped sending off résumés for college teaching positions and began to explore industrial research possibilities. He'd always been clear about not being a part of any industry or business that contributed to military purposes, and this decision was a major one. I was distressed that he would opt for just any work slot and now wondered what that would mean for all of us. In any event, whatever Mark did in the near future would have to take the availability of medical facilities into account.

He was aware, these days, of the changes in his physical appearance, and was troubled at being so "out of shape." Though it was hard for him to have lost control over his own body, he spoke with humor about his distended stomach and loss of hair. His once-full beard was sparse and scraggly now, and he said he might as well shave the whole thing off. It'd been a part of him and who he was for so long, however, that I asked him not to, and he kept it on for my sake. Whatever he might have felt about his appearance did not prevent him from continuing to teach class or interacting with his fellow students.

The days following the third hospitalization had much more of the sense of a "meanwhile" for us. We were conscious of the brevity of our other reprieves and our joy this time was qualified. We treasured whatever private space we could claim for ourselves, and early one morning when it was just the four of us in the house again and the children were still asleep, Mark came grinning to the breakfast table, in the raw. Sun patches dappled the kitchen alcove, and we lingered over breakfast, glad for each other, and for that carefree moment, almost stolen now it seemed, to be the selves we once had been.

One afternoon, before Mark went off to do some work at school, I said that there was a poem I wanted him to read. I handed him Bradford Smith's "Roll of Film"[1] from the pamphlet *Dear Gift of Life*.

Snip, snap: will it be fifteen, sixteen before the thread snaps?
How do you finish a roll death finishes first?
Take pictures of my love, of growing old, of all the tender care
  of you I had in mind, of spring and all the seasons we walked
  through together and would walk again, of places far and near,
  of youth both far yet near as forever, of books, house, bed,
  night, dawn.
Take all, take all. To keep. For you must keep them now. I
  shall go searching them in what new place and way I do not
  know, yet always here with you, with pictures or without,
  while you live out our two lives joined in some deeper,
  different way.

Live for me—live all I lack the time for:
Live double and live deep, my love.
And finish the roll in joy, nor be afraid:
It never will be finished while you live.

As Mark read it, his eyes filled with tears. He put aside his briefcase and papers and we spent the afternoon holding each other and talking about the time that was left to us. We made love, with a special tender giving and receiving of the other. As we lay quietly together afterward, Mark said he ached to think that that pleasuring should ever have to end. It was the last time we were to know each other so.

Mark had been wanting to spend some time with his mother at the home where he'd been raised. Though it was only two hours away, we hadn't been there since Mark's illness began. We made arrangements now to go as soon as Mark was freed from the daily radiation schedule. Fluid from the tumor was putting increasing pressure on the lung area, however, and by the end of the week, Mark was finding it difficult to breathe again. He had an appointment with Dr. G. on the afternoon we had hoped to get away. Dr. G. knew how much Mark wanted to get back to his old home, and he said he would do a thoracentesis in his office right then, rather than readmit Mark to the hospital. It was a lengthy and messy procedure, the drawing off of fluid from the chest cavity with tubes and needles, and a gift of time for us on Dr. G.'s part. He told Mark to call him if he had any problems while we were at his mother's and insisted that Mark see him as soon as we returned. We had until Monday morning; Mark was going home.

We'd chosen not to settle in the Lancaster area ourselves for many reasons, but now we saw the countryside where he'd grown up with new appreciation and delight. Mark spoke of it warmly, proud of the farm-lands and Pennsylvania Dutch characteristics which mark the area so distinctly. Though it was mainly a way of saluting his past, Mark wondered even then if it might be a place to live for a while after graduation.

By the time we reached his mother's house, Mark was drained and pale. The chest tap had provided only temporary relief, and he was beginning to feel the effects of the radiation series he'd just completed. Mom Albertson had prepared one of Mark's favorite meals, meat loaf and baked potatoes, but he was barely able to join us at the table. Though he made an effort to be sociable, he spent most of the time wrapped up in a large living room chair, weak and nauseated. A painful abscess developed under one of his arms, and his mother finally called her own doctor for some medication. The nighttime was even worse. He vomited a lot and was unable to lie down because of the difficulty of breathing.

Even though he still felt rotten in the morning, Mark and I went to the local bank with all of his savings bonds that had been accumulating since his childhood. He'd said for some time that he wished to cash them, in order to make that financial resource available to me in our joint savings account.

There were quite a number of bonds and Mark had to sign and countersign each one in the presence of the teller. It was an effort for him to stand, and though he struggled to control the waves of nausea, he had to stop halfway through and ask to use the lavatory. He insisted on completing the task that day.

We had made plans earlier for friends from New England to join us at Mom Albertson's home. They'd been wanting to spend some time with Mark. Herman took off a few days to make the trip now during their children's spring vacation. They called just before they arrived to check on directions and were startled to hear me say, "You've come none too soon." We'd all been looking forward to their visit. The Zinters had been neighbors and good friends when we'd lived in the inner city in Boston. Though we'd kept in close contact by phone all during Mark's illness, Herman and Carole both admitted they were nervous and uncertain of their reactions before seeing Mark now. They were all struck, especially their children, by how old and sick he looked, and by what an effort it was for him to move and breathe. His coloring was an unnatural yellowish-gray; his embrace was stiff, not from awkwardness but pain. "Not too hard," he said as Carole came to give him a hug. The signs of death were about him.

The Zinters' arrival, however, did much to liven up the household and defuse the sense of despair that had settled over us. Mark was anxious to show them things about the house from his childhood, and went upstairs, for the first time, to get out some toys that his father had made for him years before. Their son, Ansel, was intrigued by an old pair of handcuffs, and after locking him to a post in jest, Mark told Ansel they were his to keep.

Mom Albertson had prepared a marvelous roast pork meal, exactly as Mark had always enjoyed it, but he was unable to eat. Pear and peach juice were the only nourishment he could get down without gagging. He had another difficult night and sat up in bed through most of it in order to breathe. I woke around 4 A.M. to the exuberant chirruping of birds outside our window. I saw that Mark was awake and when I mumbled something about it being a good time to get worms, he burst out laughing. I awoke fully then; it had been so long since I'd heard the sound of his laughter.

The night had been so difficult, however, and the nausea so unremitting, that at 6 A.M. Sunday morning Mark finally called Dr. G.'s answering service. The doctor returned the call within the hour, suggested something to relieve the nausea, and made arrangements to see Mark as soon as we returned to the city.

Mark had looked forward to showing the Zinters the culturally and historically unique area around his home, but it was I who had to take them on the tour that day. A neighbor saw Mark's mother later and remarked, "I see that Mark came home to visit." She replied, "He really came to say goodbye."

The Zinters followed us back to our apartment late that Sunday afternoon. It was a dark, anxious trip through a horrendous two-hour-long thunderstorm. Robin and Kim both slept, but Mark and I drove in silence, Mark barely able to speak. I reached our home emotionally exhausted. We got Mark settled and opened some wine to drink in the living room. While I was out of the room, Mark spoke to Herman and Carole of his dying. He said he hoped Robin would remember him, and he talked of my remarrying, not just as a possibility, but as if to let them know that he expected it would happen and approved. Carole said later, "It was the most difficult glass of wine I've ever had."

The next day at his office Dr. G. explained the radioactive gold therapy he wished to start. The benefits of such therapy were still varied. Though it would mean isolation in a private room for several days, there were no known side-effects, and we agreed it was at least worth trying. Dr. G. told us that he had spoken to the director of student health at the hospital about monetary aid toward Mark's medical expenses and he assured us that we shouldn't be anxious about the financial aspect of the illness. When the appointment was over, I waited by the elevator while Mark stopped off at the men's room. Dr. G. came up and said to me alone, "It doesn't look good for Mark, but we'll do all that we can."

We met Phyllis, just getting off duty, as we left the hospital, and told her about the gold treatment and of Mark's rehospitalization the next day. She asked Mark if he needed someone to scream and express his

anger with, but he told her no, that he had me. The question took me
by surprise, as anger was not right then either of our responses, and I
realized how little overt anger Mark seemed to need to vent.

Herman came to drive us home. Phyllis joined us, sitting with me in
the back seat. The two of us spoke of the statistics of lymphosarcoma.
Phyllis told me that there was no history yet of any permanent remission
from it as far as she knew. I spoke of our plans for a camping trip and
said that the summer was all I was asking for now. Phyllis turned to me
and said, "I don't think you will even have that long." She had just seen
Mark's charts at the hospital. Though I was shaken by her words, it
confirmed what Dr. G. had said by the elevator, and I was grateful for
Phyllis' honesty.

Because I knew she'd tell me the truth, I asked her then what the end
would be like with lymphosarcoma, how it is that one dies, and she
replied that in Mark's case it might be by suffocation—lack of oxygen
due to pressure by the tumor on the lungs. It was a heavy conversation,
not one that Mark heard, I think. He and Herman were discussing the
university and the architectural design of the buildings we were driving
past. When Phyllis suggested a book to read now with Robin, however,
he joined our conversation, and we spoke together of the need to talk
openly with children about death.

Mark entered the hospital the next morning—round four. One of the
admitting papers had "Courtesy Patient" stamped across it; there was
to be no charge for this hospitalization. When the woman at the admitting desk routinely asked the purpose of the hospitalization, Mark told
her he had cancer of the lymph. Startled, she scoffed, "Of course you
don't. Now, don't be foolish. They'll have you fixed up in no time." It
was strange to be in the position of defending a diagnosis to the hospital
receptionist, but she was unable to receive what Mark had said. She
needed to protect both herself and us from "bad news." Mark dropped
the subject and proceeded with the business of filling out the forms.
When asked about his religious affiliation in the past Mark had always
said, "None." Now he replied, for the first time, "Quaker."

Mark was put in a four-man room for the first day and soon after we
arrived, a man in his mid-sixties entered, carrying a small suitcase. While
a nurse directed him to one of the beds, he kept fuming and sputtering

that it was all a mistake, that he didn't need to be hospitalized. From time to time, a dreadful wracking cough would seize him in the midst of a phrase, and though he announced derisively that his doctor had ordered him to stop smoking and drinking, he lit up a cigar. A half-hour later, incensed at what he felt to be a lack of medical attention, he gathered up his belongings and walked out. I was astonished at his bravado, and yet impressed by his spirited independence. Good luck to him—however he chooses to make his exits.

It was different for Mark. He had sunk into his bed with relief, and when offered the use of the nasal oxygen unit, had accepted gladly. I left him to rest, troubled now by the sight of him connected to those green plastic tubes, and remembering what Phyllis had said.

The Zinters were waiting with the children outside, and we walked around the campus pushing Kim's carriage. It was a mild April day; students lolled about on the grass. The contrast with the hospital environment was jarring, and it felt strange to have those two worlds so sharply juxtaposed in my life. Carole has said since that she was amazed by the way I handled what was happening to us, but that she also worried about that control. She knew I was depressed after taking Mark to the hospital, yet she watched me switch off those feelings to interact normally with Robin. I wasn't doing any screaming or hollering, and she wondered what I was doing with all that tension.

That evening the Zinters went to the hospital to say goodbye to Mark. I wasn't ready to admit it might be their last time with him, but it was in their minds as they entered his room. There was not much said; Mark had the hiccups and it was obvious that he didn't wish to talk much. Frustrated by a sense of helplessness, they sat quietly by his bedside. Carole gave Mark a backrub, the only way she knew then of reaching out to him. "I'd expected to be somehow more adequate," she admitted later. Before leaving, she said, "We love you, Mark." He replied, "San's the one who's going to need the loving now." There were no profound exchanges of parting words, just squeezed hands, a wink from Mark and goodbyes.

A letter and package from the Zinters arrived a few days later, with some model cars for Robin from Ansel, and wonderfully soft pillows for Mark. The letter said, in part:

Thanks, Mark and Sandi, for the time we shared.

Returning to Boston was difficult, knowing you were again eight hours away . . . The most frustrating part of the visit was not being able to offer some immediate assistance in the easing of your discomfort, Mark, and hopefully what's in the box will help . . .

If we loved you people before, and you know that we did, that love has been increased with this visit and also respect for your relationship and honesty . . .

A week later, Herman sent the following:

april now, nearly may

Dear Mark and Sandi,
both living still and that is enough
today

the night is gentle
more fragrant than yesterday . . .
and warmer:

not a small accomplishment

This common will, emerging in colors
not yet substance in the bare
but fully ladened branches:

the face of a child
smiling on autumn

my hand still in yours, firmly gripped;
and the wink across time

that is enough
today

with my love,
Herman

Treatment for Mark went ahead as scheduled. Radioactive gold was injected into his abdomen, and he was now put into a private room. He could have visitors, though we were cautioned, especially women of child-bearing age, to keep a certain distance until the radioactivity in his system had decreased. Mark rejected several offers to have a TV put in. Though he found the private room lonely and was eager to be among other people, he had no interest in the outside world that would come to him via television.

In early April, as Mark's condition became more serious, we received a letter from Becky McCall:

". . . I have been thinking of one time we all had together (I have thought of many) and this keeps coming back, with deeper and deeper sounds: We were playing a rather tedious game of 'The animal I think I am' (You saw yourself a beagle) . . . and I remember as the game became more spontaneous and we started pinning animal souls on each other . . . my eyes rested on you, Mark, and I said, surprising myself with my own voice, 'Mark is very much like the buffalo'—great giggles as the "hairy" comparison was inferred, and then the room was quite silent as I tried to verbalize the soul and Karma of the beast that spoke to the soul and Karma of Mark —and I remember a sudden flash of embarrassment I felt as I spoke of you with such reverence—that you should represent to me then, like the buffalo, such a great and tragically diminished race of man.

I think I felt too awkward and surprised by my own realization to elaborate that night, but I lived with that realization for many days—it was not long after that when Rob wrote "Quaker Soldier-Boy" that our love for you became more verbalized—and even now as we struggle against great grief to celebrate your life, we know that your life for us is indeed a celebration—and just as we feel so moved by the American Indian we have never met, and feel so clumsily guided by his profound understanding of the earth, so will our children be guided by you. You are within us forever because you have lived.

We follow this letter southward in a few days—

Our deep love,
Becky

I called them to say, "If you want to see Mark, come now."

When Rob and Becky went in alone at first to see Mark, they were stunned by his physical appearance. Mark's own ease helped their initial uncomfortableness. He seemed to understand what they really wanted to know and spoke to them directly about the cancer.

To Becky it seemed as if everything surrounding us was full of death: the littered city streets, the late winter mud, the sterile hospital atmosphere, even the ceiling tiles in our kitchen, hanging precipitously, swollen and rotten from the roof leak overhead. She was conscious of an overwhelming sadness in things not human, and constantly fought the impulse to flee. She said later that what light there was came from Mark and me—that *we* at least had an energy greater than the sadness that surrounded us.

On Friday morning the three of us went in together to spend time with Mark. The McCalls had brought along their instruments, and we sang together. Rob had written "Quaker Soldier-Boy" a few years before when Mark had been drafted and done alternative service as a conscientious objector. They sang that song now with guitar and banjo:

> Clothe yourself and shoe your feet
> Simple home and food to eat
> Enter in the States' employ
> You've become a soldier, Quaker boy.
>
> Hands are torn and knees are sore
> Be killed or slay in daily war
> Rested, tired, grief and joy
> You are of it, soldier–Quaker boy.
>
> Choose to laugh or choose to cry
> Live to live and live to die
> Freedom in the world's employ
> You have done it, Quaker soldier-boy.

They did some funny old songs, including a rendition of the McCall family "Prune Song." Then Becky, improvising a stage from a bathtowel, chair and I.V. stand, performed a number of wild animal facial mimes, including her specialty, and Mark's favorite from past years, the armadillo.

*   *   *

By Friday afternoon, Mark had been hiccuping nonstop for twenty-four hours. Exhausted and discouraged, he asked me to talk with Dr. G. to get some sense of what was happening. I went to the doctor's office and asked him for a realistic assessment. G. acknowledged that the radioactive gold treatment, which had been a long shot, was not making any significant difference; it was not affecting the cancerous cell development. "It's always difficult, with a young person, to know when to stop treatment, but I think we may have reached that point now," he said. When I asked, "How long do we have, then?" he replied, "A matter of days."

I was stunned! So soon?

Though I felt Mark should be told where things stood, I agreed to wait until Dr. G. came on his rounds Sunday morning so that we could have a longer time to talk together. I walked over to Mark's room, fighting back tears, held together by sheer will power. Though I expected him to be asleep, I needed to look in on him. I was afraid he might look as if he were dead already, but when I peered on tiptoe through the window of his door, there he was, standing by the bed, using the urinal. So much for life-and-death scenarios! I was immensely relieved to find him so obviously functioning, as if defying what G. had just said. He was grumpy and withdrawn, however, and after a few minutes, I left him to get some more sleep.

Charlie Cox, Mark's closest friend among the graduate students, was waiting to drive me back to the apartment. I told him about my conversation with G., and though he sat quietly with me in the car, I cried only a little. I wasn't really feeling any of it anymore; I was so tightly strung up inside, I was incapable of reacting. There was no release yet from the control I'd imposed on myself.

I'd been dreading the time when Mark might choose to withdraw from us as a family (known as the process of decathexis), when he might close himself off from that which still held him to this world, and I ached to think that he might not wish to see us anymore. As Becky and I folded the laundry, it was verbalizing the possibility of this loss that triggered my release. I threw myself on the bed and sobbed.

That evening the McCalls and I went back to Mark's room together. It was difficult for Mark to speak, and it was clear that he did not wish to visit. His breathing was labored and he was using the nasal oxygen unit again. We spoke little, yet there was a rich sense of being present to each other. Rob and Becky brought their instruments, and it was the universal language of music that bound us together then as it had in all our exuberant and playful gatherings in the past. Mark lay with his eyes closed in the dimly lit room, surrounded by intravenous and oxygen apparatus, his foot keeping time against the bedcovers to the gentle picking of banjo and guitar.

Rob sang another song, "Just Like I Promised," one he'd written for Mark while wondering what it would mean if what the New Testament said about life after death was really true.

> I had a dream the other day
> I saw Jehovah in a moving way
> With sweet assurance I heard him say
> It's going to be just like I promised
>   Just like I promised
>   I promised I would never leave
> It's going to be just like I promised
>   Just like I promised
>   You weren't wrong to believe.
>
> Since Moses wandered in the wild
> Since Mary had that mournful child
> I promised we would be reconciled
> It's going to be just like I promised
>   Just like I promised. . . .
>
> In shining darkness, a still small voice
> Said, You may not see it, but I've made the choice
> You've cried enough, now you can rejoice
> It's going to be just like I promised
>   Just like I promised.
>   I promised I would never leave
> And it's going to be just like I promised
>   Just like I promised
>   You weren't wrong to believe.

We were all in tears by then, Mark included. Unable to get any closer because of the radioactivity, Becky stood at the end of the bed holding on to Mark's foot. Out of the silence that followed, Mark said a kind of benediction, asking for grace for us all.

Much later that same evening, I called the doctor's answering service and left the message that I was going to tell Mark the next morning about our conversation that afternoon. A few minutes later, the answering service called back. The woman who'd taken the message turned out to be one of my neighbors, and it had suddenly dawned on her who had just called. She hadn't realized how serious Mark's condition was, or that G. was our doctor. Trained as a nurse herself, she offered now to do whatever she could to help. The generosity and concern of the neighbors on our street was one of the special gifts that we were to know during this time.

My crying woke Becky later that night, and she came to rub my back and spend the rest of the night on the bed beside me. The visit had been a good one for Rob. Music had enabled him to say what he wasn't able to say in words, and though the time had been sad, there was no sense for him of things left unsaid or incomplete. The time with Mark had been more frustrating for Becky. She'd always held a special place in Mark's affections, and the radioactivity had kept her from getting close to him. The physical distance kept her from believing it was really Mark dying in that bed, and she felt angrier as time went on that she hadn't broken the "medical rules" and hugged Mark goodbye.

The McCalls left for home early the next morning. My parents arrived shortly afterward, and I went to the hospital to tell Mark about the conversation I'd had with G. He seemed to be aware that the radioactive treatment had made little difference. When I told him we might now have only a matter of days, he said he wished it were a matter of only minutes, and that he was glad it would be over soon. In fact, if it weren't for the insurance policy benefits for the children and me, he'd just as soon take a gun and end it all now. My anguish was all the greater, knowing how he hated being in his body as it was now, yet wanting him alive and a part of us for as long as possible. I said something about his being brave, and for the first time, he became angry with me. He insisted that I didn't understand, that he wasn't brave, that the easiest thing in the world was to sit there, letting go of it all. "You're the one who has to be brave; it's living that takes the courage."

I opened a letter that had come that morning from an old college friend and read it aloud to Mark. Brad was studying in Japan, and had only recently received our Christmas and February letters. He wrote now:

> ... Your time at grad school seems to me to have put a lot of things into productive perspective. I remember your talking about your interest in urban transportation planning, and your long-time interest in computer science. I'm happy to hear you found such a good medium for pursuing both . . .

It was a heavy line to read aloud, given the realities we were trying to address that morning, and I was overwhelmed with an immeasurable sadness.

The letter went on:

> Mark and Sandi, your illness is no afterthought in my letter, though it comes at the end. My thoughts and inexpressible hopes have been with you since the night I received your letter in March telling, with more courage and understanding than I could muster in reading it, of what has come up in your life.
>
> Forgive me if in writing whatever I do here, I say things which are out of tune with whatever peace you have made with whatever stage of this crisis you are in. I do pray, with all the yearning that heart and mind can conjure together, for a good turn in things to come.

Though I had thought Dr. G. wouldn't be in until Sunday, he arrived moments later, and sat down to talk with us. He startled me by speaking encouragingly about some possible new treatments to try after the radioactivity had subsided sufficiently. When I questioned him about our conversation the previous day, he said that ethically he could not ever give up trying for Mark's recovery if there were treatments available. He did promise Mark, however, that he would not do anything that would prolong his suffering, nor would he at this point use medication that had known negative side-effects. He said he would not use extraordinary measures to add only a few days to Mark's life.

I felt confused by G.'s latest projections about treatment, and somewhat of a fool for having overreacted to the conversation in his office. Was it really not a matter of days after all? Was it possible that there still was some therapy that might turn it all around? This vacillation between hope for recovery and preparedness for death was emotionally exhausting and wearing on the spirit. One hardly dared to respond or feel at all.

When G. had gone, I opened another letter, this one from Oliver. It included these lines: "Tide-like, hope rises, falls, then rises again, while our love, like the sea, is constant."

Mark wondered then if we could ask Sue and Dave to come; he said he would like a chance to talk with them again. I called Sue from the phone in Mark's room, and thirty minutes later they were on their way to the airport. He also said he'd like to see Robb Russell, supervisor of the university's computer center. He wanted to talk about his thesis research so that what he'd done so far could be of use to someone else.

Mark was scheduled for some X-rays later that morning and I wheeled him down to the waiting area. It was a dreadful time for us. The narrow corridor where the patients were lined up was murky and depressing; the wait itself, absurdly long. Mark sat slumped in his wheelchair, weak and despondent. It was humiliating to be made to wait like objects against the wall.

Mike, our friend in neurosurgery, saw us and stopped to talk with Mark. With tears in his eyes, Mark told him that he knew he didn't have much time left, and said he hoped Mike would be able to be with him at the end.

I called Mark's mother from the hospital and told her the latest developments. Mark had said he didn't want "visitors" anymore. I told her what I understood about the process of "decathecting"—the gradual disconnecting from people and events on the fringe of one's life (casual friends, distant relations, the evening news) that sometimes helps make the final closure easier for a person with a terminal illness. It may be hard for us to say goodbye to someone we love, but the person who is dying is saying goodbye to everything.[2] Though I was sure that Mark still wanted to see his mother and me, I was trying to prepare us for that withdrawal time when Mark might choose to be freed of us all, freed of our anxiety and our caring, in order to do his dying.

Robb Russell did come in that afternoon. He'd picked up material from Mark's office at the university, and they spent more than an hour going over Mark's research and thesis draft.

Shortly after, Mom Albertson arrived. Mark said to her, "Don't think of me as this hulk of rotting flesh. My thesis is more nearly me, and my little girls *are* me." She cried openly in his presence for the first time, and when she apologized for her tears, he said, "Be yourself, Mom. If you feel like crying, cry," adding however, "only don't do it all the time —that'd be a crashing bore." He told her about having gotten mad at me that morning, and went on, "I'm not brave. I don't want to die, but dying itself is easy. I may have the pain, but San has the problems. It is she who must have the courage now, not I."

By the time Sue and Dave arrived, it had been a full day, and Mark was exhausted. I asked if we could be silent together for a little while, and we sat around his bed. We were each aware of the urgency and magnitude of the caring that had brought us together at this time. The stillness was broken finally by Mark's saying, "Thanks, friends."

Although the time we had together was brief, the quality was deep. Dave hadn't seen Mark since Christmas, and he found being with him now reassuring, as if seeing him, still alive and functioning rationally, helped to negate the idea of his dying.

We had a good last gathering before their return flight the next morning. Dave and Sue assured Mark that their home was open to the children and me if I wished to live there and return to school to get a teaching certificate. Mark was deeply grateful for that family covenanting.

As we sat together for the last time I read Bradford Smith's poem "Last Roll of Film" and then, in silence, we held hands around the bed. With tears running down her cheeks, Sue told Mark that he would never be forgotten. When Mark made some wry comment about this being a dramatic script without a hero, David replied, "Well, it sure is one hell of a cast." Dave had said earlier of our "clan" that this family was so great that "the worst thing that could happen to you would be to be the last to go." Startling us again with his imagery, Mark spoke of the death of Christ and of the importance of those who'd been with him. If no one else had been on Calvary or if no one had done anything about his life after his death, there would be little remembering of him now.

Dave knew it was probably the last time he'd ever see Mark. Conscious of the insignificance of his own trip home in comparison, he gave Mark a hug and said simply, "Have a good journey."

When they had left, Mark turned to me and said, "All I want now is to see Robin and Kim again."

CHAPTER
7
Last Days at Home

A Poem for Mark

For our own sake
we sit with you,
still as death.
My good body
denies my fear.

"I am ready," you say,
but the days keep coming
like chords
of an old hymn.

I am surprised that my question
is, How to live?
You answer it
in your dying.
Moving your body around the hurt,
You send your laughter lightly ahead
across the empty space.

—Sylvia Lotspeich
(written in the hospital corridor
while waiting to visit Mark)

Friends and letters kept coming. Dr. Carr came in to tell Mark that he and several others in the department wanted to get Mark's thesis together in time for the degree deadline May fifteenth. Although the degree itself meant little to Mark now, the time and effort needed to pull it all together at this date were substantial, and Mark was touched by the affirmation which that joint effort meant.

One of the professors Mark and I both studied with at Colby College wrote:

> I want you to know how much we cherish the memories of our contacts with you at Colby. It is not merely sentiment to acknowledge that it is young men and women like Mark and you who keep faculty members like me fulfilled in the classroom . . .

and another wrote:

> There is nothing that an aging physics professor can do or say to make your day to day life easier and happier . . . It may well be that you have more joy and happiness ahead of you than do we who feel secure.

A letter arrived from Becky:

> Your presence is constant with us. I have found that so many times, whether I'm braiding Sarah's hair, or stuffing laundry into the washer, I suddenly realize that I have been holding your hands for the past several moments—Mark, your love for us is loud and clear, and it has for each of us a personal significance that has not only touched us, but changed us. We have each grown in different ways from you—as we sing songs of you that we have not yet written, we will know even more what treasures you have left in us . . .

I wanted to bring spring into Mark's room. One day I lugged in a large potted geranium which a friend had helped me find, grinning behind its boisterously plentiful blossoms. That plant, affectionately named Alberta, is two feet high now, has produced many new cuttings, and is still going strong.

I said something to another friend one day about wanting to get pansies, a traditional part of spring planting for our family. A few hours later, she arrived on our doorstep with a dozen plants. She'd scoured the city that day, a Sunday, to find them. I took a few of the plants into Mark's room, and planted the rest in the tiny garden patch behind our apartment. It helped to work in the soil again, to show Robin how to make the roots secure and care for this new growth—to explain that in

all the cycles of nature, the old blossoms are trimmed away in order to
enable new life.

Though Mark was anxious to be transferred out of the private room,
I treasured the intimacy that the setting allowed us. We spent part of
one afternoon talking about what would happen when he died. We
talked about a memorial service, and what the children and I would do.
Mark said he'd always liked the old Fourth and Arch Street Quaker
Meeting House, and wondered if the Memorial Meeting for Worship
could be held there, even though we weren't members of that Meeting.
He hoped that friends could gather afterward to sing and eat together,
perhaps in Rosemary Marshall's backyard, since we'd always delighted
in her flower-filled urban garden.

We spoke of friends bringing homemade bread and of a favorite wine
that Rob and Becky had discovered in New England that tasted like wild
white grapes. He said then that he hoped the breaking of bread and the
remembering of our times together with friends would continue around
many tables for a long time to come. I thought we would probably go
to my parents' log cabin in New England for a while afterward, yet while
speaking of that part of the sequence, I suddenly realized I'd been
including Mark in that "we"—that I'd been picturing him in Rosemary's backyard, picturing him driving us all north later. I was stunned
into silence.

Later, between his dozings, I asked Mark if he'd like me to read aloud,
from either the newspaper or some books I'd brought from home. He
chose *Wind in the Willows*, Kenneth Grahame's classic for children of
all ages. Although attached to intravenous and oxygen units, he lay in
the late afternoon shadows of that quiet hospital room, chuckling at
favorite descriptions of Mole's spring cleaning and Rat's home in the
riverbank.

I put a new "Thought for the Day" on Mark's bedside table: "We
have loved the stars too greatly to be fearful of the night."*

I decided to go into the hospital early one morning to be with Mark
when he woke. Dressed in dungarees and an old work shirt, delighting
in the vibrancy of that early April morning, I snuck up the back stairs
of the hospital as if on my way to a secret rendezvous. Mark had just

*Exact origin unknown—an old astronomer to his pupil, Galileo.

awakened and was surprised and clearly pleased. We shared the simple breakfast tray, remembering our last "breakfast in bed" in a small Belgian hotel room several years before. For a time at least, the specter of Death stood aside, and we felt young and whole again.

When Mark said he wanted to see the children, I was determined to get them both into his room. My mother and I successfully maneuvered the kids past the guard and up the elevator. No one stopped us once we reached the private floor, and we boldly paraded past the nursing station and down the corridor to Mark's room.

I'd brought Kim in an infant recliner, and she sat waving and cooing at the foot of Mark's bed, while he and Robin put together a jigsaw puzzle that she'd made for him out of animal pictures. Mark showed Robin how to raise and lower the bed, and explained the intricacies of the call button and intravenous tubes. My mother had brought her camera, and took pictures of us—a family portrait, from a hospital bed.

Mark and I had been advised to fill out Social Security disability forms, since it was possible we would qualify for benefits if Mark's illness were prolonged. It was an arduous task—recording all of Mark's work experiences and his medical history—and I was grateful that his mind was still clear, that he was able to remember all the dates and places of employment that had paid into the Social Security system since his high school days.

Though we'd always made major financial decisions together, Mark had usually attended to the bills. During these hospitalizations, however, I'd taken over some of that responsibility, and one day I took in the large accounts book that Mark used when tallying the monthly expenses. We went over the procedure he'd been using, and he explained the filing system in his desk at home. It was easy to understand, and I let him know that I was grateful for the clear ordering of all those records. (My own desk has never been "in order"; it only gets reshuffled every January as a matter of principle.) We took time then to go over the state of our finances so that I would know what student loans were still outstanding. We'd been warned that bank accounts not shared jointly are sealed upon the death of the account holder,* so, except for the car, everything we

---

*Some states consider the male the principal account holder, and seal even a joint account if it is the male who dies!

possessed was now in my name as well as his. The transfer of car title
to surviving spouse was, theoretically, a simple procedure, so we let that
stand.

When Jim, a Friend from our Meeting, came to visit, Mark asked him
to be one of the "overseers," the small group of Friends who would help
me make arrangements for a Memorial Meeting for Worship after his
death. Jim said he would, and urged Mark to write something for those
of us who would come together at that time.

It may have seemed to others that we were overly preoccupied with
preparations for Mark's death. Yet it was for us a way of still exercising
some control over our lives. I am grateful, now, for the steps we took
then, for the clearness it gave me to go about living afterward.

For several years we'd not paid the federal phone tax, imposed during
World War II and maintained throughout the Vietnam conflict to
augment the federal military budget. Refusal to pay the tax makes no
difference to the phone company as long as the discrepancy in payment
is explained. Each month Mark would include a letter with payment of
the phone bill, explaining that the omission of the tax was due to our
moral opposition to economic participation in the war effort. Liens were
placed on our car, and money finally taken directly from our bank
account by the IRS, but it was a moral stance we chose to maintain for
the sake of living with ourselves, a response, in part, to the query of John
Woolman, an eighteenth-century Quaker, to examine "whether the
seeds of war have any nourishment in these our possessions."[1] This
month I typed the letter to the phone company, but took it in for Mark
to sign, knowing that even now he would wish to be a part of that
statement. "The most legible copy they've ever gotten," he said grinning.

A homemade book arrived one day for Mark from our niece and
nephews in Vermont. It began, "You will be missed but remembered"
and then each page was filled with drawings and rememberings of the
ways in which Mark had been special to each of them:

        for teaching me to tie my shoes . . .
        for the ride in your taxi-cab . . .
                (during Mark's Boston cab-driving days)

for fun when planting Christmas trees . . .
for help with farm chores and the wood supply . . .
for setting up your tent for us . . .
for being you . . .

The book came on one of Mark's good days, and though it was hard just then to receive such a direct acknowledgment of his dying, the pages which followed were a celebration of Mark's relationship with this family, past and future. On the card which came with it, Cil wrote,

Thanks for being a part of our lives and family.
Thanks for our two lovely nieces . . .

and Dick added,

We will do anything we can to help your family whenever help is needed. You can be sure of that.

That day also brought a letter from our friend Linny. Rather than waiting to say how much Mark meant to them at a memorial service, Linny's letter and the outpouring of love from family and other friends were "flowers" now—a way of "giving a cheer" while Mark was still here to hear what they were cheering about.

That evening a classmate of Mark's came into the room with three other fellows from the university's barbershop quartet. They asked if Mark would like a rendering of their repertoire, and before long, the room was full of ambulatory patients from up and down the hall. Their first selection was "I Feel a Song Coming On." Then they sang what happened to have been the theme song for a backpacking wilderness-encounter trip that Mark and I had helped lead two summers before, "Today."

We sang along with them, a rush of memories accompanying that song. Tears flowed freely down Mark's face, and I had trouble getting the words out. The quartet hesitated, startled by our reactions. When they'd finished, Mark explained why the song had been so special for us. He then asked them to repeat the first song, and he sang with them. It was a splendid occasion.

*   *   *

Mark had been asking Dr. G. to release him from the hospital. We both understood that the medical world had done all that it could, and that he would be going home for the last time. We talked about what that would mean for us as a family, particularly about the importance of allowing life in our household to continue in a way that was not oppressed or stifled by an aura of sickness. When we'd moved into the apartment two years before, we had decided to use the front room with its sliding doors as Robin's bedroom. Mark's and my bedroom, then, had to be the room connecting the living room and kitchen. Though it meant being in the flow of household traffic now, we made the decision not to disorient Robin by changing rooms and to allow her to play without having to be hushed up all the time.

There were practical arrangements to be made. I knew I would need help as Mark became increasingly bedridden. Phyllis and Vicki, both nurses and neighbors, volunteered. I spoke with the director of Family Services at the hospital, and she told me to let her know if we needed additional assistance. I also phoned the Cancer Society to make arrangements for the use of aspirator and oxygen units when they became necessary.

The morning that Mark was to be released, Dr. G. sat down with us to discuss medications and procedures for modifying pain. I took elaborate notes, glad to be entrusted with that aspect of Mark's care. The nurses had gathered up supplies for us to use at home, such as the plastic urinal, surgical scissors and tape. Our doctor friend, Mike, had told Dr. G. that he would be available to help us at home at the end, and we knew that we could call on Dr. G. whenever necessary as well. Mark joked about getting back with his favorite roommate, and our conversation with Dr. G. was light-hearted. Mark seemed stronger and in better spirits than he had been for a long time. Though we were aware of the implications of this trip home, it was a victory to be going home at all, and there was for both of us a kind of exhilaration, a sense of adventure about being on our own again for this next phase of our life together.

That first evening at home, Mark said he'd like to see some of our Ugandan pictures again—not those we usually showed to groups, but the personal ones. As we looked at them together, I realized that there would never be anyone else to whom those pictures would mean as much; Mark was the person with whom I had shared that unique experience. Years from now, when old pictures might be brought out for grandchildren and adventures recounted, I would be doing that telling alone. I would have liked to work our way through all the slides, but we'd hardly begun when Mark admitted that he wasn't feeling well and needed to lie down. I offered to set up the projector in the bedroom, but Mark had no energy even for that. I packed the pictures away.

Though there were to be only seven more of them, the days, as Sylvie wrote, kept coming "like chords of an old hymn." We settled into new patterns of being a family. Mark ate little and slept a lot, yet he seemed glad to be among us. Robin would stop on her way out the back door to show him her latest drawings, and she lay on the bed between us while I read her nap and bedtime stories. When Mark took a bath, Kim sat in her recliner on the bathroom floor. They held unintelligible cooing conversations together. At first he dressed each morning, and took charge of his own medications, but he soon spent more and more time in bed, and it was I who kept the medication charts.

He woke me once at dawn to listen to a woodpecker, incredulous that such a bird should be there in the city for him to hear at all. We got up then, and had some tea together in the quiet of the kitchen, the door open to the early rays of the sun. The house was full of blooms these days, pussywillow and forsythia at first, and then later, apple, cherry and lilac blossoms.

The nights were the worst for Mark. He was wakeful and uncomfortable, exhausted by the struggle for breath as the tumor continued to grow. When the pain became too great, he would wake me to ask for more medicine. He was amazed, he said, at my ability to get up then, responding out of a deep sleep, when he could hardly lift his head. It was good to have him next to me again, yet I ached to see him in such distress. I was still getting up to feed Kim during the night, and afterward I would often read aloud until Mark dozed off. Caring for him at home was a way of putting the love to work, and I was glad that there was something I could do. The hardest time for me was the early morning after Mark had dropped into a troubled sleep, and I lay awake beside him waiting for day.

These last days were a time for preparing Robin for the future. I had talked with her before about the seriousness of Mark's illness, but I explained now that he might not ever get better, that in spite of all that the doctors had tried to do, her dad might die. We read children's books together which discussed death (though there were only a few of them then): Miska Miles' *Annie and the Old One* and Judith Viorst's *The Tenth Good Thing About Barney*. As we worked in the garden, or as I threw out wilted blossoms, I talked about the life and death of all living things. When we found a dead bird in the backyard, it was examined and talked about, and then buried. I consulted my pediatrician. He felt that though there were many developmental theories about children and death, she should take her cues from me. "If she sees you cry, she'll know it's okay to cry, and when she sees you laugh again, she'll know that that's all right too."

On his second day home, Mark was speaking about a friend of ours when he suddenly said, "He's the only eligible guy I know of who'd be right for you." I was startled by the topic and unable to respond. Later that afternoon a friend of a friend called to say that he'd be glad to be of assistance to our family in any way he could. I'd never met him, but knew that his wife had died several years before. He gave me several helpful insights about familial tensions from his own experiences and ended with the suggestion that we get together sometime. Painful and confusing as the future seemed, I *had* begun to wonder what it would hold for *me*, and this conversation with an eligible stranger was intriguing. When I turned to Mark, his eyes were filled with tears, and he said in a strangled voice, "I hope I get to meet the guy." He admitted he was feeling jealous already, and then began to vomit. I ached to think that that conversation had caused him distress, and I was torn again by the conflict between death and ongoing life that surrounded us.

Later that evening, Dean Jones—chaplain, ethics professor and friend whom I'd first met when I spent my junior year at Fisk University— called from New York. He'd counseled us before our marriage, and with Oliver, had performed our wedding ceremony. He said something now about "paying his debts"—about affirming Mark's and my place in his life. He had had no way of knowing how much worse the situation had become since our February letter to him—it was one of those providential connectings.

We were continually reminded of the caring of others. The McCalls put together a tape of favorite songs, including some funny ones especially for Robin and Kim. Mark's aunt sent canned goods and food supplies via Mom Albertson, and a neighbor arrived one morning with a large box of paper plates, napkins, cups and canned drinks.

Oliver came again, this time with his wife, Eleonore, and a family friend, Emily. The brevity of the visit and the physical constraints inherent in our apartment were difficult aspects of their time now with Mark. The position of his bed in the flow of household traffic, and the number of people who passed through that particular day, made it hard for Oliver and Mark to have any real quiet time together, something that Oliver missed. Mark had not suggested changing his physical surroundings, though once when the rest of us sat talking in the living room, he asked if we couldn't all come into the bedroom instead. We sat around the bed then, some of us on the floor. It wasn't that he had anything specific to say; he'd simply wanted to be included in the conversation of family and friends.

There was no pretense or denial among us; Mark was as forthright as ever. He spoke to Eleonore of his sense of waste at having to die so young, and Eleonore said later that being with us that day was "like staging a play, where the only real character was Mark."

Mark had an appointment with Dr. G. that afternoon, and for the first time, admitted the need for a wheelchair to get from the hospital entrance to the doctor's office. The examination seemed fairly routine, but when we reached home, Mark could barely stand, and Oliver and my father had to carry him between them up the front steps.

A woman from our Meeting, who lived on the other side of the city, arrived bearing a pot of lentil soup for our supper. A few hours later, she appeared again with more soup. When she'd seen how many there were of us, she'd gone home and made another pot. The Powells and Emily left after supper, Em offering to use a week of her vacation later in May to help us if we needed.

Though Mark still had spells of nausea, he seemed stronger by the weekend, getting dressed and out of bed. On Saturday morning, a friend picked up a wheelchair for us from the Cancer Society and brought it to the apartment. We rearranged the furniture so that Mark could get around in it more easily. At first he was like a kid with a new toy, "varooming" around the corners with Robin in his lap.

I knew he couldn't manage much effort on his own for an excursion yet, but I was full of plans for taking him places with the help of the wheelchair. We'd always wanted to hike an old stagecoach road along a creek that led to a little inn in the woods. I began to make plans to do that trail with Mark in the wheelchair some early morning, arriving at the inn for breakfast and connecting with friends afterward for a ride home. I was determined to get him back into the natural world. Out of the medical environment, it seemed reasonable that he should get well again. Irrational as it may seem, I was expecting him to get better; I wasn't ready yet for him to get worse.

That Saturday we went on an outing to some land the city had conserved. My father drove with Robin in the front seat; Mark and I in the back. I was delighted to see the magnolias and Japanese cherry trees dripping with blossoms, but I often turned to find Mark with his eyes closed, beads of sweat forming on his ashen brow. Dad drove to our favorite kite-flying place, and Robin rolled and tumbled down the hills, coaxing her grandfather and me into various games of hide-and-seek. Mark got out of the car but remained leaning against the fender for support. Another car pulled up and a man emerged to exercise his several dogs. I came upon the two men discussing breeds and habits of animals, and wondered at the effort and conscious will it must have taken Mark to carry on that conversation.

When the man and his dogs left, Mark got back into the car, anxious to head home. Dad and I carried him between us up the front steps and barely got him to the room before he had another siege of vomiting. The trip had taken more of a toll on him than I'd imagined, and though he claimed it was worth it, I wondered now if he would ever be able to make another.

On Sunday morning we had a "called" Meeting for Worship at our house. Mark was in no condition to get to our regular Meeting place, so I'd asked for a special Meeting to be held in our own home. Mark insisted on getting dressed, and sat in the wheelchair in the living room. My parents and Mark's mother were with us that day, and Friends from our Meeting soon filled the chairs and floor space of the room.

It was Mark who offered the first message. He said he'd been thinking of all the young men and women and children who were dying right then because of the Vietnam conflict. He spoke of the love which supported him now, and of his distress at the indifference with which human beings in that other land were being destroyed by our country. If only we as a nation could care about others as he knew himself to be cared for, then ways could be found to resolve conflicts between peoples without war.

It was a "gathered" Meeting, messages arising out of a deep communal silence. One Friend, conscious of Kim's gurgling in the background, spoke of the paradox of being present as a man's life drew to an end, while the life of his child was just beginning, yet he reminded us that most of the people who have ever lived are dead now (a mind-boggling thought, even now, for me). A Friend whom we'd met in East Africa remembered that when she'd been brought to our home for the first time, we'd said the Ugandan welcome, "Kuli kio" ("Come in"), and that our lives had been saying it ever since. Another said that the flight of wild geese, touching our lives, sometimes only briefly and then moving on, was now and would continue to be a reminder for him of Mark's life. My father, who does not easily share his emotions in public, waited until the Meeting was over and then, with a full throat, thanked those good people there, Friends and friends, for their support of our family.

Many who spoke to or about Mark that day were not to speak later at the Memorial Meeting for Worship because their affirmation of his life had already been given, in Mark's presence. I said that morning that it was a cause of celebration for us, not only to realize that Mark would be mourned after he died, but to know, so clearly now, that he was loved while he lived.

Later that day, a good friend stopped by to see us before taking off for a week-long conference. As she left, she said to Mark, "See you next week." Aware of a different timetable, he replied, "Goodbye, Fritzi."

Sunday evening my parents left for home, but Mom Albertson stayed on to help us in the apartment. Mark's condition worsened. By Monday, the left side of his face had begun to droop, pulling down the eye muscles and allowing him only a curious half-smile. He admitted that his vision was blurred now, and we realized that cancerous cells might have begun to affect the central nervous system. With Dr. G.'s consent, Vicki and Mike came to the house to perform a spinal tap, a test to determine whether the cancer had metastasized to the brain. It was an awkward and difficult procedure, Vicki kneeling on our double bed in order to help Mark maintain the necessary position. Though it must have been very uncomfortable, Mark never complained. Though I wonder now why we bothered with that test, I'm sure we did it then because just the knowing of the medical facts gave us a handle on reality.

Monday evening Mark was violently ill before he could get to the bathroom. As his mother and I helped him back to bed, he said how grateful he was to be taken care of. Robin brought her special bedtime blanket and told him he could use it. Later that night, Mark experienced sudden sharp pain for the first time, and during one trip to the bathroom, blacked out in my arms. Mom Albertson and I took turns rubbing his back throughout the night. He asked now for heavier doses of the pain medication that Dr. G. had made available, determining for himself how often and how much of it he needed.

He said at one point, "I don't think I'm going to make it to next Christmas, Pooh," and then, with disgust, "Shit, I don't think I'm even going to make it to my thirtieth birthday"—five weeks away. "What a bloody waste."

That afternoon, May 2, we heard that J. Edgar Hoover had died. At Mark's request I phoned a number of friends to say, "Mark Albertson is pleased to report that he has managed to outlive J. Edgar Hoover." For one who'd lived through the FBI harassment of the sixties and early seventies, it was an accomplishment for Mark.

There was little sleep for any of us that night. Mom Albertson alternated with me as we talked or rubbed or read Mark through the hours of pain.

On Wednesday morning, he told me where he'd filed the title to the car, and read to me what he had written so far for his memorial service. I'd hoped he might write something special for the children as well, but he was never to get to it. The film in our camera had one exposure left, and Mark took a shot that morning of Kim asleep in my arms. Then he explained the intricacies of changing the film, and sitting in his pajamas on the edge of the bed, taught me to reload the camera.

Mark had an appointment at Dr. G.'s office that afternoon. I realized I would need help getting him there, and called his friend Charlie at the university to ask if he could come with us. He said he'd be there as soon as possible. Mark struggled into a shirt and trousers, but when he was done, he lay curled up on the bed on his side, gasping for breath. Almost inaudibly, but with a clear sense of urgency, he told me then that he wanted to go back into the hospital, that he had to have help with his breathing. Though I was dismayed at the thought of another hospitalization, I had no other way of relieving his distress at this point.

I called the police, explained that my husband was dying of cancer, and asked for a rescue vehicle with an oxygen unit. I phoned Dr. G.'s office next and left the message that I was bringing Mark into the emergency ward. Charlie hadn't come yet, and panicking, I called Mike.

Gusts of rain pounded against the windows; the house was dark inside, heaving with our silent, helpless waiting. At last the doorbell rang. Two policemen stood in the foyer with an assemblage of tanks and hoses. Dripping water from their black slickers, they followed me down the hall into the bedroom. They put an oxygen mask over Mark's face and turned on the machine. Mark's gasping continued, and his whole body strained with the effort to take in the oxygen.

Mike arrived a few minutes later, and in seconds realized that the oxygen unit was not working properly, that it was, in fact, costing Mark even more energy to breathe than without it. Somewhat abashed, one of the policemen called in to headquarters to ask for a replacement, but Mike suggested getting to the hospital as quickly as possible. Since it seemed absurd to expect Mark to sit up in a regular car, we decided to risk the journey in the police van.

As I followed the stretcher outside, I met Charlie just coming up the stairs. Only later did I learn that he had had no car when I'd called to ask for his help, and he'd alternately run and walked, fifty steps at a time, the fifteen blocks to our house.

Neighbors stood in their doorways, silent concern on their faces. Mark's stretcher was laid on a side bench in the van, and Mike and I climbed in next to him. The paddy-wagon doors were shut, locking automatically from the outside, and we drove off.

Robin stood at the window watching our departure. Two years later, I was to come upon her holding an old flowerpot over the nose of a stuffed toy. When I asked what she was doing, she explained that she was a nurse giving oxygen to Doggie who was dying. It was the last image she had of her dad.

The First 365 Days

May 1972

Dear Friends and Relations,

This letter I write alone. There were five hospitalizations and numerous, only temporarily successful, courses of treatment since it all began in December. With quiet dignity and a knowing, accepting mind, Mark died the evening of May 4th.

We had both hoped he could be at home at the end, but because of internal hemorrhaging and difficulty breathing, Mark decided to be hospitalized. When it became clear that transfusions could not help, Mark asked that the heroic measures be stopped, so that he could finish his life without the intravenous apparatus, blood pressure readings, etc. The morning of the 4th, all previous medication was stopped, and morphine begun—to relieve the pain and enable the "letting go" process.

It was a "good" day (if that can be understood)—filled with quiet sharings, sleep, laughter, singing (even a rendition of Rob and Becky's prune song). Early in the morning we delighted, not so much in the breaking, as in the transcending of a hospital rule. Kim was "snuck" in under a dear friend's poncho, and as I nursed her by Mark's bedside, we had a deep sense of the continuum of life. As the day wore on, the dozing and incoherent ramblings increased, but in and out of it all was clear recognition of persons in the room, sharing of ginger ale and brownies, a comment on Robin's drawings, and a treasured description of the texture of whole-wheat bread. Death came about 7:45 in the evening. There was, for me, only an immediate glad acceptance that he had been released from suffering. It was clear to me that his spirit was no longer confined to a physically troubled form, but freed to go a new and different way. As he wished, his eyes were given so that another might see, and his body donated to medical research. . . .

There has been through this whole process an awareness of how much a part of life death is. To accept the certainty of one's own death, whenever or however it may occur; to see oneself, finally, as a part of a larger whole, related to all of the natural process, is ultimately freeing. There was for us no sense that Mark's death was an act of God. We do not worship a whiskered gentleman in the sky who wills that mine shafts collapse or school buildings burn or young parents die of cancer. We may grow through suffering, but I do not believe that we are made to suffer in order that we may grow . . . We accept our place within the laws of nature and willingly "take our chances in this vast splendid creation . . . The gift of life is inseparably united to the promise of death; on no other terms is life ever given." We do not ask that either the heights or depths of life be otherwise. Whatever the pattern of our lives, we are sustained and upheld at the core of our beings. Someday the puzzle of cancerous cell growth (ironically a matter of too much life) will be understood and controlled by medical science so that men need not die of that cause so young. To think that it is within man's power, now, to stop the death of young men sent to war— that is the greater tragedy. . . .

One real cause for celebration for Mark during these last months was not so much the knowledge that he would be mourned after he died, but the very real knowledge that he was loved while he lived. The time between January and May was for us a grace period, a gift—a chance to live deeply and openly with the knowledge of death, and to have made real to us the love and caring support of those around us. Speaking freely of death enabled us to taste more fully of life. . . .

The three Friends that Mark had asked to help me with memorial service arrangements came over the evening after his death and we talked about the Memorial Meeting for Worship to be held on Sunday afternoon. Word went out about the celebration that was to be held afterward at Rosemary's house, and I began making whole-wheat bread. The logistics of travel and housing were worked out somehow, and people started arriving.

I met Mark's mother at the Meeting House. She was wearing a bright

yellow and black outfit that Mark had especially liked, and together we
greeted friends and family. A large piece of parchment for people to sign
rested on the table in the entranceway. It read: "Gathered May 7th,
1972, at the 4th and Arch Street Meeting House to Celebrate Mark's
Life." I was amazed at the number of people who kept arriving, more
than a hundred and fifty, and was touched by the distances traveled and
inconveniences overcome in order to be with us that day.

Many who came up to me before the service were visibly pained and
needed to share their sorrow. It was not a time of tears for me, however,
but rather a celebration and a giving thanks for Mark's life as we had
known it. I was high, glowing with all the love and support manifested
by this coming together of people.

There was no sense in me that day of sack cloth or ashes, no wailing
or dirge. Perhaps for some this way of addressing a death seemed strange.
Funeral pomp and circumstance is appropriate and necessary in many
cases—but there was no casket and no laying of Mark's body in the earth
this day. Mark and I had planned for this together, and it proceeded out
of where Mark and I had been and where I was now. I had already done
much of my immediate grieving. The long haul was still ahead, of course,
but unlike an unexpected death, I had been preparing myself for Mark's
death. Because we had already done some of the grieving together, the
journey toward healing had begun as well.

The seating arrangement in the Meeting House was semicircular,
with a small table and single facing bench in the front. A family friend
had brought fresh apple blossoms from her backyard, and we placed
them in an old earthenware crock Mark had found as a child. They were
the only flowers; the newspaper death notice asked that contributions
be made to the American Cancer Society or American Friends Service
Committee instead. May apple blossoms are still for me a most lovely
and difficult part of spring.

I chose to sit with Robin and Kim in one of the first benches along
the side. I wanted to be able to see those who had come to share this
time—not with my back to them. When the children became restless,
a friend took them outside, playing hide-and-seek among the rhododen-
dron.

As in all meetings for worship, we came together in silence. One of
the overseers rose after a few moments to explain the nature of Friends'
worship, to affirm that we were gathered now out of thankfulness for a

life known and shared, and to encourage friends to speak out if they felt moved to do so. I stood then and read the message that Mark had written for this day, something he'd done that spring and given to me the last day he was home.

> To friends gathered here and scattered everywhere—peace. Some of you have asked me to write something for this occasion, to express how I feel it should be. I can only try.
>
> We make a very special thing out of death . . . and in some sense this is fitting—death does often seem final.
>
> But I see death as an instant in time, like birth, between two very different types of life. We celebrate births; let us celebrate my death. We don't have a good name for what happens after death; but the life which has come to a physical end, because it has been lived, continues to affect the lives of those that have been touched by it.
>
> Then let this be a time for us to examine our lives and our life together . . . to resolve the grief and re-rejoice about happier times.
>
> So as this celebration continues and enlarges during the next hours and weeks, let us blend what tears there may be . . . with tea, and Kleenex with cookies . . . for richer lives.
>
> In a very special sense, I am with you.

There were silences between the messages, difficult times, perhaps, for those struggling with whether or not to speak. As the time flowed, the sense of the Meeting deepened, the silence and the messages offered releasing other messages. As a "gathered people," we shared laughter and song and tears.

One of Mark's professors spoke of what Mark had taught him about life, and a young doctor who'd been with us throughout spoke of how much he had learned from Mark in those four months. Emily read lines from Auden's "In Memory of W. B. Yeats," and Sue, the passages from Paul Tillich[1] and *The Velveteen Rabbit*[2] about being real that she'd written to Mark in a letter that he never saw.

> In his *Eternal Now* Tillich writes that "nothing truly real is forgotten eternally, because everything real comes from eternity and goes to eternity."
>
> Then I think about what being "real" means and I remember

what the skin horse tells the velveteen rabbit—that you're real
when someone loves you. Perhaps Tillich would have said it differently, but I'm sure the meanings are close.

Mark, you've got to know that you've been loved, really loved,
by quite a few people and that makes you Real and never, ever to
be forgotten.

We're thinking of you and loving you a whole lot.

Carole Zinter shared her son Ansel's response that Mark was a good
man and should have lived to be a good *old* man, and my sister Cil told
of their nine-year-old's statement: "I hope Uncle Mark is having fun
with God" and of how that fit so well with their sense of Mark's zest
for life. My brother-in-law Dick spoke—all the more special for his usual
Vermonter's reserve—recalling a day with Mark thinning out cedars to
make fenceposts and allow room for other trees to grow, adding that
Mark had a similar effect on others' lives, his life helping to make new
growth possible for others.

Rob McCall sang "Just Like I Promised" and later in the hour Mark's
mother stood to explain that Rob had written it for Mark and asked if
he would play it again so we could sing with him. What a relief it was
to sing, tears streaming down our cheeks. Sometime later Loey Powell
asked for Rob's guitar. It was passed along the bench behind me, and
then she stood and sang "Hurry Sundown," its lyrics reaffirming the
peace that Mark had made with his life and death.

That time together was filled with love for Mark—and admiration for
the way he'd lived and died. My heart full, I stood at the end of the hour
and gave thanks for that time together and for those people through
whom Mark had known he was loved while he lived. It was, strange as
it may seem, a splendid occasion. Professional mourners we were not.
It was like a great reunion of the best of friends, and Mark's spirit was
so present among us that there was not yet a sense of loss. Loving support
and affirmation in such condensed measure was a high for me. One
friend said later that I'd looked radiant that day, almost bridelike. In
contrast, the sadness on my twin's face presaged what was to come for
me.

Almost all of us went then to Rosemary Marshall's house. Her daffo-
dil- and wisteria-filled backyard was a spot Mark and I had always

enjoyed. Surrounded by the city, it offered a quiet "secret garden." White-clothed tables were covered with breads of all kinds—whole wheat, buns, stollen, braids, all homemade. Some friends made bread for the first time as their offering for that day; one loaf was sent down from Boston by a family that couldn't come themselves. Butter and honey pots, wine and cider made up the rest of the feast. When it seemed that everyone had gathered, I shared with them Mark's hope that such a breaking of bread might go on around many tables for many years to come.

I wrote to friends a few weeks later from Sue's home, where the children and I had gone to spend the month:

... And so—what now? Robin and Kim and I have been scooped up by our family . . . The dying process Mark and I could at least partially share, so it was easier for me then. The hard part comes now when I so much need his strengths. There are lots of really hard moments—at dusk when Mark would be coming home for supper, when I think or read something that I want to share with him, when Kim does something new and delightful that he would have rejoiced in, when Robin asks, "Who'll make mountains (knees to slide down) for me now that Daddy is dead?" and all the unguarded moments when one is torn apart anew. Sometimes there is no comfort—only tears and deep aching and the passage of time.

Yet the healing process has begun. The pieces are fitting into new places, new designs. The "extended family" is a good thing. There is much laughter and deep quiet caring in this household, and I am kept whole by the living that goes on around me. Kathryn (5) says to Robin, "My daddy will be your daddy now that Uncle Mark is gone." The little ones help fill my days, along with bicycling, batiking, attending Friends Meeting here in Oak Park. Life has a way of pressing on—I spent the evening a week after Mark's death on a peace march, carrying a candle for him, for his spirit was with us as surely as his body would have been. Dear neighbors here have brought in meals, held garage sales to help pay for our plane fares, studied up on Quakerism and sought out ways to know more about Mark and our style of life together. So, too, the sum of remembrances keeps growing. They are now the channel for

Mark's love, as his spirit and the quality of his life continue to touch and inform ours.

To all of you, I would say (as I'm sure Mark would wish me to): Live out your love for one another now. Don't assume the future; don't assume all kinds of healing time for the bruised places in your relationships with others. Don't be afraid to touch and share deeply and openly all the tragic and joyful dimensions of life.

And the future? What can one say, for sure, ever again? I'm leaning on an old Quaker saying, "Proceed as way opens." Mark had such a sense of the ongoingness of life that I feel I must honor it. I'm exploring the possibility of working for a Master of Arts in Teaching degree. There are good M.A.T. programs in the Chicago area, and Sue has offered to care for the children while I do some more studying. That may be a real way of putting the year "in trust." While it would be hard to leave our old home and the support community there that has shared so with us these past months, a grace period to prepare more securely for the future makes sense. We'll see.

And so, dear people, thanks for *being,* for holding us so deeply in your caring . . . for countless meals brought in, for geraniums and apple blossoms and all the others signs of spring's rebirth; for opening your homes for friends from out of town, for *coming;* for songs, and poems; for washing dishes, and providing paper plates; for errands run, and quiet standing still. In subtler ways, the caring continues and is returned, across all kinds of time and distance. That, at least, is for sure.

Much love,
San

My family urged me to close up the apartment completely and go to Chicago for a year. Much of the future hinged on my getting into graduate school in that area, however—a mind-boggling process in itself —and I was still unclear about whether to move out of our old community permanently. I needed time to think before pulling up all our stakes, and I decided to leave final plans for later.

I used Sue's gentle presence to go through the rest of Mark's things —his closet, the winter clothes already put away, his desk. It helped to have someone to do it with, someone who had also cared for Mark, for whom some of the clothes had a history as well (like the jacket he'd worn when we all went to cut the Christmas tree).

I kept a number of old work shirts for myself, but gave most of the rest to friends. Rob still wears a vest I'd made for Mark that Christmas, and it's nice to see favorite old ties appear again on Oliver or my dad.

Mark's body was to be used for medical research during the coming year, the cremation and burial of remains of all the donors that year to be carried out by the Anatomical Gift Board at some later date. There was a memorial service now which Mark's mother attended, held at the Chapel of the Four Chaplains, itself a memorial to four clergymen of different faiths who'd given their life jackets and their lives that others might survive during a sea disaster. I was glad she could be present to see her son acknowledged among this company of others who had given something through their deaths as well as through their lives.

There would be difficult times for me throughout that year—living with the knowledge that Mark's body was still among us, that some young medical student was studying it, the mole on his shoulder, exposing his muscles, veins, sinews; knowing in a radically intimate way that physical form that I had known with a different kind of intimacy. I knew that that body was not Mark now, that who he really was was somewhere else, freed from that physical form, but I had loved his body too, had known and been known by it, and I hoped now that in this final task, before it was returned to the soil, it would be handled with care and skill and some appreciation for the life which it had nurtured.

I was sent Mark's diploma. His thesis material for his master's work in computer science had been put into publishable form in time for graduation. Fellow students had organized the writing, and the chairman of the graduate group, Dr. Carr, released his personal secretary from other tasks in order that it could be typed in time. It was an act of generosity and respect for Mark. Word also came that the corneal transplant performed after he died had been successful, another dimension to the ongoingness of life.

There were aggravating, energy-consuming hassles with life insurance agents, death certificates, bank account notification and car title transfer, and it was at least a year before all the paperwork was finally completed. It was incredible to me then that at the time when one has least energy to deal with such matters, one is subjected to the most typical bureaucratic hassles and runarounds.

I'd already sent a copy of *On Death and Dying* to Dr. G. and Mark's surgeon. Now I baked bread and returned to the hospital with it to thank the staff for their care of Mark.

I knew I needed to walk those corridors without Mark, to connect with those people again—to help me not to hate hospitals or the medical world forever. I had spent so much time there in the past four months, attending to Mark's needs, that I had to go there this time to get perspective, to claim the territory where the focus of my grief had been most real, to own the reality that Mark was no longer there.

I'd feared it might be awkward and uncomfortable, but it was not. Dr. G. was warm and gentle. We talked about some of my plans for the future; he urged me to keep in touch, and we parted with a hug.

It became clear to me at last that spending a year in Chicago at graduate school, living with Sue and Dave, would be the right thing to do, and I closed up the apartment. On the day we were to leave, a young girl from across the street came to the door. With an awkward "Us kids are all sorry you're going," she thrust an envelope into my hand and fled. It was filled with assorted nickles and pennies and love.

We drove to Mom Albertson's for a brief visit. It was an important stopover psychologically. Though Robin didn't say so directly, I sensed that she was hoping Mark would be there and needed to check out each room before she could lay down that possibility. I had never been in this setting without Mark, and both his presence and his absence were immediate and real. Evidence of his life was all around us—clothing in drawers, an old wool shirt in the hall closet, mementos from his childhood, things he'd made in this home for his parents, and articles from Uganda that we'd stored here.

Now almost all of our belongings from the apartment were here as well: our washer and dryer, books and boxes lined the walls of the basement and garage. Memories and dreams intertwined, came to rest here, the material things of our life together gathered again at this place of his beginnings. With our two children and a half-dozen cardboard boxes, I was about to begin another chapter of my life. I sat on the cellar steps and wept.

Before going to Chicago, we spent some time at my family's log cabin in Sturbridge, Massachusetts. Medical crises seemed to follow one after the other: nausea and dizziness for me, chicken pox with secondary infections for the children. There were days when I had only enough energy to feed and diaper Kim. She was still nursing— the only satisfactory mothering thing I seemed able to manage—and we spent a lot of time in the rocking chair together. All too often I was unable to respond appropriately when Robin whined or fussed or displayed feistiness, leaving it to my mother to discipline or soothe or distract her.

I found that the more removed I became from Mark's illness, the less acceptable was his death. The cabin with surrounding woods and lake were awash with memories of Mark chopping wood or sailing, of our having breakfast on the beach or making love on the cliffs behind the cabin. My raging began in earnest.

The film which Mark had helped me load into the camera was finally sent off for developing, and I eagerly awaited what I knew would be the last picture of him, taken when he'd come to sit with Robin and Kim at the breakfast table his last morning at home. The photo, when it finally arrived, was devastating, and I was caught off-guard by the truth it revealed. Though it captured a reality with which I'd lived only six weeks earlier, I'd already managed to forget how Mark had looked then, how sick he really was. The photo was almost grotesque now compared with the woodsman image I'd been remembering lately. Yet both were real depictions of Mark, and acknowledging that duality helped me put his death into perspective again.

To my amazement I found that this was not to be the "last picture" of Mark. Friends, some of them out of touch for several years, sent snapshots now of Mark from earlier days—photos I'd never seen, some from camping trips together, some even from his childhood. One was of Mark reading to the children during a visit to the Vermont farm, Robin and her cousin on his lap, others clustered about the chair. It had been taken two years earlier, the neglected film only now discovered and developed. So the connectings went on—others' memories of Mark bearing witness to his life as a whole.

I found myself compulsively going over the details of Mark's illness with friends, though often without emotion. What I really needed was to talk about Mark's life and to have others remember him with me and with Robin.

For some, however, even among my family, there was a silence about Mark, as if they thought of him as a chapter in my life that had ended now. Perhaps they hoped to spare me the pain of remembering, as if not talking about it would help me not to feel the loss. It is hard to mourn among others for whom life goes on as usual, and it is hard for others to have a mourner in their midst.

Since the accepted rituals of mourning end so abruptly in our society, the continuation of one's grieving just feels awkward to others. Mark's mother's grief, deeper in ways other than mine, was different, and we could comfort each other only obliquely across the distance. In spite of the good people about me, I felt very alone, solitary in my interior work of grief. I was given tender hugs and pats, but there was no one to hold me as I needed to be held.

For friends one of the most devastating parts of Mark's illness was the realization that it had happened to one of their peers. So many within our circle were at a similar stage in their lives—seven years of marriage, young children, the culmination of academic study and the beginning of careers. With Mark's death came the specter of mortality for us all.

While they did not grieve as I did, there were friends who helped me do the mourning that was mine to do. A few days after the memorial service, Becky wrote:

These are the difficult times coming on—more tears than tea right now. You have sweet memories that are only yours, and the inevitable emptiness that goes with them. It was painful to leave you on Monday. I felt that if we could all only stay together and face *together* the reality of Mark's absence, it might be easier, but that's not exactly "carrying on," is it? There is for you grief that we can never touch—but we will "tend to the garden" while you remain inside—and we never ease our embracing of you even as we must leave you alone. There is hope in healing. Grief will move in and out of every moment too quickly, too immense for you to touch or contain—it may for a long time—yet someday, the morning will feel full again, and Mark, like some giant cypress in your memory, will stand still. This is the hardest time, and you are dear to me . . .

Another instance of friends offering succor came a few weeks later, when the children and I were visiting the Bings. For a while, it seemed that Robin might have appendicitis. Though it turned out to be only stomach cramps, I felt it was too much to handle. I curled up to rest that afternoon in a sleeping bag on the Bings' family room floor. Barbi put on some music and then went upstairs to care for the children. The music triggered in me such a depth of emotion and sense of release that I began to cry. All the tension of holding myself together—all my efforts at being a composed mother and daughter—collapsed, and I sobbed and sobbed.

Barbi heard me and came downstairs. She sat on the floor beside me for a while, rubbing my back and stroking my head, and then, without speaking, went quietly away again. With no words of rhetorical comfort, no pat phrases or professional jargon, she gave me that day what I needed most—a "screaming room," a place to wail, to do the raging I could not do in my own parents' home, for all their love and care of me, and I was immeasurably grateful.

The music I heard that day was Johannes Brahms' *A German Requiem,* a touchstone for me now.

> Blessed are they that mourn for they shall be comforted.
> —Matthew 5:4

They that sow in tears shall reap in joy.

He that goeth forth and weepeth, bearing precious seed, shall doubtless come again with rejoicing, bringing his sheaves with him.
Psalms 126:5–6

I wrote in my journal that summer:

> simple disbelief sometimes—
> inconceivable not to see him again
> missing wing-tucks—talking in the night
> someone to complain to
> hard—finding recipes that want to share
> remembering Uganda—
> who'll speak Luganda with me now?

wanting him to see R. and share in her growing up—

when will there be joy in the morning again?

who will ever love, care about my body
          the C. section scar going down

wanting—fiercely—for him to know things
          believing—if it's important for *him*
               that he know those things,
               then he already does—

          does this world matter to his spirit now?

          he lived in it so fully once—

hard to find things with his handwriting—
          a list of gifts to Kim—begun while I
               was in hospital

hard days—these
          flood of bright aching memories

hard to realize—no more gifts from him
               my birthday coming—
          no more gifts for him—
               yet finding things I would love to give

My journal was filled with troubled indecision about our family car. Should I trade in the microbus? There were such emotional ties with that vehicle. I pored over *Consumer Reports,* feeling like an idiot. It was to be my first major business transaction as a woman alone. How to keep from being taken, ripped off? Wanting to use the life insurance money wisely; hassling the incorrect car titles, negotiating the papers. How not to be "the pathetic widow"? The relief in realizing suddenly that this change in cars now didn't mean I could never again have a car that easily carried canoes and kids . . .

Midsummer was spent on my sister Cil's dairy farm in Vermont. They were good cathartic hours for me—pulling weeds in the garden and lifting bales from the wagons. I lay on new sweet-smelling hay high in the barn loft, watching swallows, drinking in the sunlight, mending—and wept there one night through a howling thunderstorm. I visited friends nearby and met a woman married now for the third time, her life full of tragic losses, yet resilient and still capable of loving—a good lesson for me.

My niece and nephews prepared a special memorial service of their own for Mark, planting and dedicating an apple tree in his honor. They read a poem, about the transitory beauty of blossoms, and played a recording of the song "Let there be peace on earth, and let it begin with me." I found my nephew, nine, weeping on the stairs afterward. "Why did Uncle Mark have to die?"

Back in Sturbridge my self-image hit a new low when Sue and Dave and their children arrived to spend time at the cabin. Robin seemed so difficult and demanding, and I felt rotten as a mother compared to my sister. I had no energy or initiative, and found it hard to keep up even my part of the chores. I felt bloated beside my twin in her bikini, and disliked myself inside and out.

We went to a housewarming one evening, a family gathering to celebrate Oliver and Eleonore's new home. Too late I realized I'd forgotten a gift. Would I ever get past my own pain? I was so conscious of Mark's absence, which no one else seemed to notice anymore. I knew I was using others, was dependent on their energy, yet I couldn't seem to manage any differently. I felt guilty about being such a basket case, but I couldn't seem to break out of my self-pity, that draining, numbing sadness. I was grateful for the nurturing of others, yet so tired of having to be grateful. What had happened to that composed, centered person who'd been so strong during Mark's illness? Where was that part of me now?

In August we held a covenant celebration for Kim, as we had for Robin, celebrating her birth and covenanting to hold her in our care. A blessing for Kim offered by Oliver asked not that she be spared "danger or risk or dark valleys, but that she know the courage to face such things undismayed."

"Way opened" for the fall. I was admitted with full tuition to the Master of Arts in Teaching English program at the University of Chicago, and the children and I went to live with Sue and Dave for the year. I had a sense of beginnings again. Some of my own choices were at work now: graduate study, a new car and a new home.

A few weeks after our arrival, Sue and Dave made plans to have a family outing on their own. For the first time since Mark's death, I was to be alone with my children for a whole unscheduled day; the three of us would be "a family" on our own, and I approached the day with dread.

I knew I needed to get us out of the house, so we headed off for a small Friends' Meeting a half-hour away. It was a clear bright autumn morning, and memories of similar days with Mark came flooding back. I missed two expressway exits and cried most of the way there while the children slept in the back seat.

During Meeting someone spoke of the mistaken view of fall and winter, of all the death imagery usually associated with those seasons, when really it is at that time of year that the essence of life is found in its most intense form—condensed within a seed. I thought of Robin and Kim, the ongoingness of Mark's life in them, and was reminded of something Mark had said near the end of his illness. "There are signs of life in all seasons; you just have to look harder sometimes."

After Meeting, the children and I drove to a nearby arboretum for a picnic lunch. We walked around the lake, Kim in the backpack, along one of many miles of trails. Robin and I collected leaves and acorns, and investigated the underside of old logs, and a gladness grew in me that I had not thought possible. It was our first expedition, just the three of us. I wrote in my journal that night: "We did it! Onward!"

A photo arrived, from a college friend of Mark's—autumn milkweed, the new seeds poised, ready for flight; and a few days later, a sketch of an autumn leaf from Herman Zinter, surrounded by these words:

10/29/72
alone, late on Sunday afternoon

I stirred the fire embers which were not felt, and
set a record turning which was not heard,
having left the warm room for day's end outside.

> standing on the stone steps looking beyond to discover
> this was my thirty-sixth autumn in thirty-five years.
> some can look forward to twice as many, unknown to them.

Mark knew twenty-nine, or less, when,
     during an inversion of seasons,
   passed, while spring green and an infant daughter were new.
quiet, except for droplets falling on wet leaves
    (drizzle is not heard, only slightly felt),
and rubber tires on wet asphalt, four times each passing,
     single file, two ways.

brilliant red this leaf: part of shrub over shoulder's height;
    orange berry; branch with ridges
high leaf falling
to that spot!
where will it be next spring?

Course work went well at the university. I found my mind being
stretched in ways it hadn't been for years. A whole part of me that had
been laid aside when I got married was being tapped again; I was being
affirmed academically and professionally, and it felt good. Since no one
there knew Mark or my children, I was only me. Influenced, enriched
by all of their lives, to be sure, but here, essentially, and existentially,
myself.

Yet it was strange to be back in the singles' world. On the application
forms, one is classified as either married or single. I knew I wasn't
married anymore, but I certainly didn't feel single. I wondered what to
do with my wedding and engagement rings. What did they symbolize
now? Keeping them on my left hand was a kind of protection, a definition of myself that I was familiar with. It gave me someone to be until
I could find out who I was aside from Mark's wife. By thus signaling my
unavailability, I could also pretend that it didn't matter if no one found
me interesting or attractive.

Yet I was available, and hungry, not so much for involvement as for
the security which I had known in a loving relationship. I really didn't
have the energy for intimacy with someone else, but I wanted to be
taken care of again.

I resented the "meat-market," "looking-over" process, yet was guilty
of doing the same to the men I met. It was almost a relief when I'd spot
a characteristic that would "disqualify" someone from being an acceptable spouse or father, for then I could just be friends. It was an ugly,

tunnel-vision approach, this baggage I carried into human relationships. I wore a huge "Feed Me" sign emotionally, yet was terrified of exposing myself to the risks of intimacy, to the fear of rejection and the possibility of loss again. What a nest my marriage had been, to know myself loved and respected and desired. Where were the props now—to trust my own self, my own worth?

I finally realized that it was foolish to wonder what to do with my rings. When I stopped feeling married to Mark and felt different about myself, then I would be able to change them to my right hand or take them off altogether. My own inner reality would provide the signals for the outer symbols.

There were still many hard moments for me, days of living close to the surface of myself. I went with friends to the symphony and wept through most of it, the dark and ethereal passages echoing timeless emotions of pain and release.

There were times when I wished that I'd wept more with Mark and had let him know how much I would miss him. My strength then, almost stoical, seemed absurd now. Yet I knew that our actions then had their own integrity: we were as we were, and did what we did. We could not have cried or held each other enough then to have eased this pain now. One never says it all or finishes with the loving. Perhaps my not knowing at the time Mark was dying what missing him would *really* be like later made it possible to get through the experience. How good that we do not know all that is ahead—that we do not have to live out the future in the present, that both the pain and the healing come in their own time.

Being an extended family had its own special fullness—learning the margins of others—living in a home that was not our own, helping children deal with the sharing process, having someone with whom to get the car towed, pick out Kim's first Christmas bear. It was not an easy year for Sue, caring now for four children instead of two. I was getting applauded for graduate work, but one gets little stroking these days for increased mothering, and the space between my sister and me often wore thin. We each remember that year differently, with different pain; the healing of it only now, with time, and the sense of a new history between us.

There were good heart-easing times—center-ring seats at the circus, *Godspell* and Chicago Bulls games. One of my classmates, a Dominican sister, became a special friend. We had a common base for spiritual questing, mysticism for Quaker and Roman, and a delight in Charlie Chaplin, William Faulkner and a "little glass of something" after exams.

Spring arrived, bringing its own ache and rememberings. Jonathan, now three, asked if Uncle Mark was in the ground with all the worms and mud.

I rose early those days, baking whole-wheat bread to send in little loaves to those who'd been with us the year before; kneading the dough, a way to work out the anguish as memories came back in waves.

There were many who remembered with me. Phyllis wrote:

Just a quick note to tell you that I am thinking about you and rejoicing in Mark's life . . . I hope this next year will bring you fulfillment and renewal. Please stay in touch. I treasure the time we had together.

And from my aunt:

There is so little that anyone can say, only that we all care, and I love you. Mark was such a fine person in many, many ways. We all miss him.

The next Sunday the Downers Grove Meeting House was filled with apple blossoms.

CHAPTER
9
" . . . Because I
Need a New Daddy"

This is the place where Daddy is dead—
with flowers all around.
Where is Daddy's body? You didn't take me there yet.
—Robin, age 3 1/2

Robin began to ask to see where her dad was buried, so on a trip back to Pennsylvania that next November, we went to the cemetery for the first time. I called the Anatomical Gifts office and was startled to learn that the burial of those remains that included Mark's had taken place only the week before, eighteen months now since his death.

We found the cemetery in one corner of a ghetto section of the city, a curiously juxtaposed area of grass and trees surrounded by neglected apartment buildings and an expressway. A small sign along the trash-strewn street marked the entrance: PERPETUAL CARE—NO PLANTINGS PERMITTED.

The annual burial sites for Anatomical Gifts are designated by flat numbered markers, and we finally found the section along a back wall. A rough, uneven patch of freshly turned earth faced us, the square marker resting among jagged chunks of broken glass. It was bleak and desolate, and I knelt among the clods of earth and wept. Robin squatted beside me, silent and thoughtful. When I asked her some time later about that day, she remembered "Just sitting there, being quiet for a while. I knew you were crying, Mommy."

. . . he only paused, quitting the knoll which was no abode of the dead because there was no death . . . not held fast in earth but free in earth and not in earth but of earth, myriad yet undiffused in

every myriad part, leaf and twig and particle, air and sun and rain
and dew and night, acorn oak and leaf and acorn again, dark and
dawn and dark and dawn again in their immutable progressions
and, being myriad, one . . .

—William Faulkner, "The Bear"

We'd collected a few sprays of autumn oak leaves and acorns before we
came, and stuck them in the earth now next to the marker. We went
back, for Kim's sake, when she was older. New grass covered the glass
by then, and the children played hide-and-seek among the old tomb-
stones nearby. I have no sense that Mark is there.

I've wondered about the effects of the loss of a parent on the lives
of my children, about the scars that that experience leaves, about what
I could have done to have made it easier.

The one thing I wish I had done differently is to have given Robin
another chance to say goodbye to Mark, to have broken the rules and
gotten her into his room somehow that last day, as we did with Kim.
There is no way of knowing what difference it might have made,
whether the fact of death or the loss would have been any easier to bear,
and the wishing and wondering need finally to be laid down. I've missed
Mark for my children; I've missed for them the father I knew they did
not have, the fathering they would not know. Yet I realized I must
separate my own sadness from their experience of that loss, and not
project onto them my personal pain. From the beginning Robin seemed
to understand more about death than most theorists claimed was characteristic or possible for three-year-olds. For the most part, she understood
that Mark was not coming back, and her missing of him was openly
expressed. She'd remark suddenly on a color that matched her dad's
bathing suit, or recall a time when we'd all gone for a walk in the woods.
As I tied her sneakers one day several months after he'd died, she said
unexpectedly, "I 'member Daddy dancing with you."

That first summer she often asked to talk about Mark rather than be
read a bedtime story, and we would take turns remembering different
things he'd said or done. Lugging a rocking chair by herself onto the
porch, she would comment, "My daddy was a good helper." She often
asked to read aloud with me a book by Rabbi Earl Grollman, *Talking*

About Death,[1] in which the name of the person who has died is inserted, anxieties talked about and questions answered.

For many months Robin did numerous drawings of the four of us. A year later, she started to draw a picture of Mark to send to Mom Albertson, but became frustrated and angry, saying she couldn't remember what he looked like. The offer of a photograph to help only made her more irritated, and she finally drew a hippopotamus instead. Later, she brought me a drawing of a circle. "It's empty," she said. "A dead person . . . my daddy."

Although she stated crossly once that she didn't miss Mark, Robin admitted later that she was really angry at him because he'd died. She needed repeated reassurance that Mark had not wanted his life to end, and later she told her cousin, "My daddy wanted to stay and stay and stay." She would often say she wanted to see Mark again; it was hard for her to realize that that could never be so. As I tucked her in the night of her fourth birthday, she said, "I wish Daddy could have come to my party." The inequity of it all troubled her, and she announced crankily that she didn't see why she shouldn't have a father if I still did. At supper one evening she said she wanted her father, and then, with some bitterness, said, "He left us all alone." That same night, as I tucked her into bed, I got her to talk about all the people that Mark had known would help take care of us. At the end she added, "And there's somebody we didn't even see yet—a new daddy."

The desire for a new father wove like a contrapuntal theme through Robin's grieving. A month after Mark's death, she announced, "I want a new daddy, cuz I *need* a daddy." Part of her concern for a new father had to do with her awareness of *my* sadness: "I be happy when we get a new daddy. Then you won't miss our old daddy . . . When we get a new daddy, you won't ever be sad again, won't ever cry . . ." as well as her own need. At age five she said, "Oh, I wish so much I had a daddy so he could help me find a birthday present for you—cuz last time no one helped, so I just made you a picture."

Grieving in a child takes different forms, and Robin's needs and sense of loss were expressed in a variety of ways. Once a bright, merry child, she was more withdrawn, subdued now. Her moods swung rapidly from playfulness to dark sulking. Her infections, tummy aches and other complaints during the next year were often signals of a need for more attention from me in the midst of my busy academic schedule. She knew intuitively, as children often do, where adults' vulnerable places are. She learned she could trigger a sympathetic response simply by saying she missed Mark. There were times at first when she was being scolded when she would cry for Mark, protesting that he would allow her to do or have what she wanted, and I had to help her understand that her dad would have felt the same as I about the way she was behaving. On a different occasion, it was she who called *me* up short, when I misused Mark to make a point. My nephew was brandishing a measuring stick as a gun and I said, "Uncle Mark would be cross," whereupon Robin chirped, "He can't be cross, because he's dead."

She would sometimes invent stories of things that she and Mark had done together. It seemed important to me to help her keep the truth separate from her own fantasies so that we could remember and celebrate those things which had actually happened.

The release of tears came for Robin during the night. She would often wake sobbing, "I want my daddy." Her deepest outburst of grief, curiously, was not triggered by reference to Mark at all, but by a television dramatization of the Passion story the spring she was four years old. She responded to the account of Jesus' death with tears of such anguish that they revealed a very immediate and personal pain.

Once at the supper table, she suddenly asked, "Mom, do you think Daddy remembers us?" How to comfort her, how to hear what she was really asking, without offering a theological treatise. I answered with what was real for me at least: that I believed that even though her father's body was dead and buried, his spirit was with God and his love for us continued. That seemed to be enough.

Although at first Robin asked questions like "Will Daddy come up again out of the ground the way chipmunks do?" her subsequent attempts to explain death to other children indicated an understanding of its permanence. Two months after he died, Robin said, "When Kimmie is growing up and asking where her daddy is, we'll tell her Daddy is dead and we won't ever see him again."

After seeing the film *Charlotte's Web* Robin wanted to know: "What happens to animals when they die?" and "Why don't dogs live as long as people?" I explained that their bodies wear out sooner. She was quiet for a while and then said: "I know what lasts the longest . . . the world. *It* keeps on going; new people are being born all the time, even though some people die. If nobody died, there'd be people everywhere, wouldn't there?"

Just when it seemed that I'd finished working through all these issues with Robin, I was caught off-guard again by Kim. She came into the kitchen one evening when she was two-and-a-half. As she sipped a glass of milk, she suddenly asked, "Where did my daddy go?" and it hit me that I had to go through it all with her again—the explaining, the comforting. I told her that her dad had died of an illness called cancer. "Oh," she said. "But he loved you very much," I said. Kim replied, "No . . . died. I didn't hardly even have a dad."

Kim was only two months old when Mark died, so she has no memories of him to respond to or grieve over—only an awareness that she does not have in her life a father such as she sees in other homes. When she was only two years old, however, she understood the tones of sadness and mourning. Without knowing its title, she heard Richard Strauss's work *Tod und Verklärung* ("Death and Transfiguration") on the radio, and said, "That music make me sad. I wish my daddy would come back." Her images of Mark now are those which we have shared with her through stories or photographs, and I am especially glad for the pictures I took of him holding or caring for her during those last months.

Her play activity has often included a father. She would "make cakes for Daddy" in the sandbox; "I'm making believe I have a daddy and he stays here." When she was four, she told of a dream in which she went "through the woods and came to a tepee. Daddy was inside sleeping and he came home with us. But it wasn't true, because Daddy died, didn't he?" At nursery school when the paint ran down a picture she was doing of me, she labeled it: "Mommy crying when Daddy died."

I heard Kim whisper into our aging dog's ear, "I love you, Manda, and I don't ever want you to die." She spent a lot of time examining a dead squirrel along the road and we talked about the difference between being asleep and dead. She doled out M&M's one day when she was almost four:

KIM: One for Kim and one for Robin, and one for Mommy and one for poor little Daddy—I wonder what he's feeling?

ROBIN: He's not feeling anything.

Manda did die, a year later, several hours after being hit by a car. We had left her at the vet's for the night, expecting her to survive the accident. When she died, I asked the doctor if we might see the dog one last time. Having left her so hopefully the night before, it was important now to see her so clearly without life. The children stroked her head, and felt the stillness—the "dead weight" and the coldness of her form. We stood quietly holding hands around the table on which she lay, and then each said last loving words to that dear old family pet. In the spring we buried the cremated remains in the woods in Sturbridge, planting partridge berries and mosses to mark the spot.

One day, at age six, obviously distressed, Kim told me that she'd been thinking about "when there's nothing of me anymore." Though I know now that these feelings are common to small children, regardless of whether there has been a death in the family, it was hard for me then to understand that she should have such thoughts so young. We talked about the anxiety many people feel about death, and I shared my belief that there is a part of us called spirit which does not end with death; that the love and care of God that we know during this life continues in some form when this life is done. Kim was quiet for a while, then said, "Maybe Daddy's spirit is coming into a new person being born," and hopped out of bed to start the day.

> Be sure and tell them, from this father, that their father loved them very much . . .
>
> —From a letter by John Carr,
> chairman of Mark's graduate group

We've done a lot of remembering together as a family, part of the time-binding, storytelling process. I've asked Mark's mother if she would put down her memories of her own childhood and Mark's, and she's recording and writing stories from her past for us. The children and I have talked about the things we used to do as a family—the hide-and-seek game where we finally found Mark under the covers in Robin's crib; the time he let Robin play hairdresser, and the barrettes discovered still in place after he'd been out walking the dog; his presence at Kim's birth; his diapering and bathing of them both; the "mountain slides" made of his knees; Robin's trips with him to his office at the university; family hikes.

The summer after Mark died, Robin found me crying upstairs. Though she was only three, she sat quietly with her arms around me. "Do you want Daddy? I want him too." At last she went and got all her blankets and a favorite book, *The Best Nest,* one she'd memorized from the retelling, about two birds who get separated, lose their home and are at last reunited. She "read" it aloud to me for comfort. When I thanked her, she said, "I can always do that for you when you get sad."

And yet she fears my dying now as well. "What if you die while Kim and I are still little?" I can't deny that I will die sometime; I can't promise that I'll always be there. Yet I have told them that I have every intention of living to be an old lady, of being a grandmother to their children, and we have talked about the people who love and would care for them if anything did happen to me. The children know that legal arrangements have been made with Sue and Dave. I've finally updated *my* will and set up a trust fund.

Part of our bedtime ritual includes talking about the day ahead— making plans, explaining where we'll each be. It is, for us, not so much a claiming of control over the events of another day, but a reassuring sense of our place in it, and a trusting in the strength and wisdom and care which will see us through it, whatever happens.

CHAPTER
10
Three Is More
Than Four Minus One

Dear Friends and Relations,

Since September, the children and I have been renting half of an old two-family house in Concord, Massachusetts. We have five tiny rooms, an upstairs/downstairs, guest room with sleeping bags (so come), a large garden area, skunks, a duck pond 100 yds. away, a hungry oil furnace and no insulation, a negligent landlord, lots of sunshine, and an apple tree next door. In spite of all the hassles (I'm waiting for the tow truck right now), it feels really good to have our own home, and it feels good to me to be able to make it so.

A workshop with Elisabeth Kübler-Ross this past summer on death and dying marked an important point in my grief work. Learning about the pain of others provided a kind of bridging out of my own experience, and the week brought a clearness about my desire to work with others, whether in a classroom or seminar or hospital, sharing the "lessons which the dying have to teach the living about the quality of life."

I wrote my Master's thesis during the fall—a high school curriculum unit on the treatment of death through literature and language arts (film, music, drama, fiction, poetry); mailed it back to Chicago, and got the MAT degree a few weeks ago.

The end of the thesis-writing brought with it a kind of "postpartum depression," but I don't lack for things to do. I'm in babysitting and food co-ops in the area, and have joined a local chorus (doing Haydn's *Creation* and *Carmina Burana* in the spring). The kids and I go into Cambridge Friends' Meeting on Sundays, and I'm a part of a small "meeting for searching" that gathers once a month in each other's homes. I'm learning to play the guitar, trying to finish late Christmas presents (including a highchair for Robin's doll), and I still haven't done Wednesday's dishes.

I've been tutoring and leading workshops on Death and Dying at hospitals and schools in the Boston area.

If we can manage it, I'd like to spend some more time at home with Robin and Kim right now, rather than take on a full-time job. Managing carefully, we can get along on Social Security survivors' benefits (Thanks, FDR). It means tight budgeting (recycled clothes, day-old bread, homemade gifts), but the simple living has been the righter path for us anyway.

There are lots of times when it's difficult being an only parent, trying to meet the needs of two little ones. Suppertimes are still hard. Robin sees other Dads coming home and says she wishes hers was too. We mourn him now, though, in quieter ways. We are close to dear friends and family, and when I reach my margins, we often pack up food and jama-bags and arrive on their doorsteps for a "holding."

There is yet to be, for me, real joy in the morning. That will come, I'm sure, with the sharing of life again with another. Having known that kind of wholeness, I wish it to be so again.

In all of our meanwhiles, dear people, thank you for your special care of us.

The driveway is shoveled. Come break bread with us.

Love,
San

So we began the process of establishing the new home for the three of us. This task was eased by the supportive people in our neighborhood. We've swapped garden produce and child care, and car-pooled whenever possible. The concept of the self-contained, self-sufficient nuclear family will never work for me again as an adequate model of home life; the whole network of life shared with community has taken on new meaning for me.

It was a time now of discovering and defining who we were as a family. Though we continued to miss Mark, we were more than just "four minus one," and we began to build ways of being with each other that could claim wholeness for ourselves.

Our days hold much that is good: family traditions—Halloween donuts, May baskets, picnic breakfasts by the duck pond, night walks when the moon is full; Quaker family camps during the summer, a work project helping to build a solar house for a school in North Carolina, a trip with Mark's mother to the Canadian Rockies to meet relatives. We do a lot of reading aloud, especially at mealtimes, of children's classics and old favorites *(Wind in the Willows, Winnie the Pooh, A Wrinkle in Time, Little Women)*. We do not feel ourselves a "fragmented" or "fractured" family. We're able to claim who we are rather than grieving for what we are not.

I've had to come to terms with the fact that I cannot be both parents to my children; nor should I ask that they be more than children to me. I was tempted at times to treat Robin and Kim as peers, sharing thoughts and feelings with them because they were *there* and the person I used to confide in, have weighty discussions with, vent anger on, was not. Yet children cannot, and should not be asked to, take such a place in the world of adult feelings, and I needed to weigh carefully those issues appropriate for them to know of, and find other outlets for handling those which were not.

I've had to find ways to balance my own needs with those of the children, allowing time and space for myself, without feeling guilty— careful not to lose my self in the mothering of my children. Though our financial resources were slim, some extras were possible, and each year I bought season tickets to the Boston Ballet or the symphony. I audited courses at Harvard Divinity School, to continue my interest in contemporary theology and ethics, and substitute-taught in English at a nearby high school. A special gift of money, and the decision that it was all right to spend it on myself, made possible a two-week backpacking trip through Scotland, to visit English friends from Uganda days and spend a four-day retreat on the island of Iona.

I was ready now to lay down the role of "the widow." I stopped speaking and leading workshops on death and dying; I became tired of talking about my own experience, tired of being the resident resource on mortality.

Part of the ceiling hangs loose in the back hall, revealing stairs which lead up into a previously unknown, undiscovered section of the house. The stairs are steep, narrow and winding, lined with antique miniature dollhouses and old tin toys. I see everything through tones of sepia brown—as in an old photograph.

The rooms upstairs are furnished as in the 1800's—beds, dressers, closets, all left as if suddenly abandoned; a white, collarless shirt still lies on the bed. I explore room after room until I enter one that is small and bare, with wooden walls. The floorboards on which I step drop away suddenly, and I find myself in a dark airless pit.

Feeling about with my hands, I discover I am surrounded by bodies—dead, some still fully clothed—former occupants of this upper "house," as if they too had been taken by surprise in this room.

I experience neither horror nor fear. Working in the dark, I drag the bodies into the center of the space, piling up the corpses and loose bones. By standing on the top of this pyramid, I am able to reach the trap door above me. I push the boards aside and climb out. I am free.

—A dream

No one person has an edge on suffering. I'd known the love of a good man, a good marriage. Perhaps it would not be so for me again soon, perhaps not ever. Some have not known even that much. My own sadness and longing could be lived with; I didn't want to feed on self-pity or bitterness. Some kind of peace could be made with that space in my life, channeling the energy, the loving, into other relationships. I remembered a message offered in Meeting:

Embrace loneliness, and it will become solitude . . . and found that solitude could indeed be a time and space for listening, deepening— discovering who I was, besides alone.

> how to keep from getting wrinkled inside?
> > brittle, insular—a closing off
> > emotional atrophy
> how to keep alive the willingness to risk, trust,
> > be vulnerable again?
> having learned to manage on my own—
> > how not to miss the possibility of a
> > loving relationship?
> > how to keep from being blinded by self-sufficiency,
> > limited by my own resourcefulness, independence?
> do I have to be forgiven for the strengths
> > on which I have learned to draw?
> > > > —journal

I had plenty of needs of my own, wanting to love and be loved, to be affirmed physically as well as emotionally, yet it was not an "aside" or an interlude I sought, not the position of "the other woman" in some secondary relationship. I hungered for sustained relationship with someone who valued family and long-term commitment. I had to determine for myself now, in this new age, on new and different grounds, how deeply to share outside of marriage. I have known the love and care of good men since.

There have been endings for me as well, the pain of loss, disappointment, misplaced trust—more devastating in some ways than loss through death itself; days of self-doubt and unresolved anger turned inward, eroding my sense of worth. It has been a time of testing for me, of realizing when I have lost my "center," have gone afield from what is right and integral for me, of discovering that which brings joy, and that which does not. The learning and growing go on. It feels good to be clearer about what I seek in a loving relationship, to be at peace with where I am. The longing for life with another exists alongside a clear sense of claiming that which is good in my life now. The tension between "making it" on my own and wishing to share life is a tension with which I have learned to live, proceeding as way opens.

> self-respect—
> a needing to belong
> to oneself first
> happiness—a by-product
> not a goal to be sought for itself
> good deep-down sense of pleasure
> in being me—
> gladness of heart
>
> —journal

The "bread" continues to be broken, around many tables—the sum of remembering, ongoing. There has been, for me, a real sense of harvesting—a process of enrichment which has moved through and beyond the experience of loss itself, of celebrating the covenant between Mark and me and the way it worked out in our lives. I will get over Mark's death; I don't have to get over his life. Part of me shall always love him, our life together irrevocably a part of my own history now. Mark was my best friend as well as husband, lover, father of my children —and I miss him in my life. I have learned, however, that though I was enriched and extended by him, by the quality of life as he knew and lived it, yet I am not defined by him.

While any experience of loss holds in it the terror of abandonment, I have learned that we are each, finally, essentially, alone. I cannot ask that anyone else always be there for me, to fulfill me or make me happy; I cannot ask another to be responsible for the measure of my own worth. Whatever spark it is that gives meaning and validity to life is an internal one: the peace sought, inward. My essential definition is not dependent on relationship with another person, but on that which is of God in me —that spirit, that Light, within whose infinite love and amazing grace I stand.

These sheaves are brought in with rejoicing.

Part II

SHEAVES

1
Intimations of Mortality

Most of us proceed, I suspect, as if we believed personal mortality to be an unfounded rumor. Our culture is comforted by the illusion of the "twelfth good fairy," who assures us that the little princess will not die when she pricks her finger, but merely sleep for a hundred years. We have become good at insulating our lives, creating an outwardly death-free, youth-oriented culture that removes our dying to hospitals and nursing homes, and our dead to be repaired to give the illusion of life in funeral parlors.

Nature's daily interweaving of life and death, once so obvious to a rural agrarian society, has become distorted by our present-day urban settings and cultural attitude toward death. Our capacity as a nation to wreak destruction on others (Hiroshima, Vietnam) is matched by our need to develop elaborate defense systems. Television and movies are so saturated with violence that most adults and children are no longer touched by the deaths that parade nightly across the screen. Heroes blown apart one evening reappear a few days later in a new series. We either deny death, or treat it so callously that the value of life itself is eroded. We find it difficult to conceive of the possibility of genuine ending.

Our culture has, in large measure, turned to our physicians, our researchers and specialists, to serve as our theologians. It is from them that we expect perfectability and miracles. We assume that all medical problems are solvable; as if, given an adequate understanding of heart disease or malignant cell formation, the medical world will find a way to eradicate death itself. We count on our doctors to diagnose and cure us—even of our mortality. Is it any wonder that they sometimes play God, that they see death itself as an affront to their profession, that they feel their failure to provide immortality is a violation of their Hippocratic obligation to sustain life?

We must free our physicians to be human, and ourselves to understand the limitations of human knowledge and skill. We need to admit the place of death within the life cycle. In spite of all the expertise and efforts of the medical world, death is a part of the human condition. Its place is not limited to the closure of old age. Twelve-year-old princesses die, and so do twenty-nine-year-old fathers.

2
The Myth of Protective Silence

How does a physician or a family decide how much to tell a patient, how do they determine whether truth is too painful? This issue of "truth-telling" is often a central one for family and medical personnel working with patients diagnosed as having a terminal illness. The issues are complex, and there is no universal answer. Speaking the truth as one understands it is always limited by an imperfect knowledge of the truth as a whole. No one can determine for another how to respond, for each person's dying is as unique as each life.

In most cases the lines of communication involving a terminal illness are between the doctor and the patient's next of kin. It is expected that conferences on the patient's condition will be held out of the patient's hearing, and it is in the corridors outside the room that the real information is conveyed. Usually the family in dialogue with the physician determines what the patient will be told. Often, "for the sake of the patient," the decision is made to withhold the actual diagnosis, and the family and medical personnel slip into patterns of pretense, building up an intricate façade that claims things will be okay.

The decision "not to tell" may be an attempt to protect ourselves, a defense against having to admit that our loved one is, in fact, going to die. We often project onto the patient our own reactions, our own anxiety about death, our own sense of helplessness at being unable to stop the suffering.

I believe it to be a gross injustice, however, to prejudge a person's ability to cope with difficult information. We are all complex human beings, capable of a wide range of response. Though someone may become depressed or angry or dismayed at learning of his terminal illness, that does not mean that that person is incapable of coming to terms finally with the illness and proceeding with the unfinished business of life. Those who would withhold the truth for fear the patient will "fall apart" oversimplify the nature of human response.

I do not believe that it is the prerogative of anyone—family, physician or clergy—to deliberately withhold medical information from a person who has gone into the hospital or into surgery for the express purpose of determining his condition. I feel so strongly about it for myself that I'll come back and haunt the person who tries to keep the truth about my own body from me.

There is a big difference, however, between diagnosis and prognosis, and in the ways by which that information can be conveyed—between offering medical facts and telling someone he or she has only three weeks to live. The important point is to *offer* the truth and to allow the patient the freedom to accept or reject it. The way the truth is told and the kind of support that accompanies it are essential to the quality of the response on the part of the patient.

Is it even possible to keep such knowledge from another person? I suspect that most people know when they are close to death. We are, after all, an organic part of the animal world and not so out of touch with our physical selves that we do not know when our systems are in deep trouble. How could we suppose that the patient senses nothing, receives no signals!

In addition to interior signals, there are those given off by people around him. The patient can detect artificial cheerfulness and is not insensitive to the maneuverings of family and physician. Hospitalized and confined within four walls, his sensitivity to surroundings is intensified into an acute awareness of the dynamics, particularly the interpersonal ones, of what goes on around him. Glaser and Strauss's book *Awareness of Dying* discusses the variety of ways, subtle and not so subtle, by which the truth is communicated—all the ways hospital patients discover the nature of their illnesses.

What a patient does with the self-knowledge or the revealed knowledge is another matter. There are people who consciously or unconsciously deny the fact of a terminal illness. That is their right. For some, this reaction of denial is a "coping mechanism" used until such time as enough internal resources can be gathered to handle the information directly. The human mind is perfectly capable of rejecting, filtering, reconstructing, reinterpreting the data it receives, temporarily or indefinitely.

The real danger of trying to protect by silence is that the patient may wish to share his own reactions to the illness. Yet one of the greatest fears of a person with a serious illness is abandonment. In order to protect himself against desertion, the patient may participate in whatever façade is necessary to keep from being deserted by those who cannot address the truth.

Thus the protective silence becomes itself a form of abandonment. To deny a person the chance to talk out concerns and anxieties is to deny that person's deepest self. It further isolates the patient at a time of great emotional stress. The pretense weakens his self-esteem and works to destroy whatever control he might still have over his own affairs. Far from reassuring the patient, the pretense further alienates him from those he cares about and from whom he might draw strength. Mark's despondency and withdrawal and my own anguish at the way we were handling his illness were signals—though we did not recognize them at first—that at least for us there had to be a better way—a way for us to deal with Mark's dying that was more consistent with the way in which we had proceeded with our life before.

More than anything else, protective silence is a waste of quality time left together. Our responsibility should at least be to refuse to perpetuate a myth that can be the obstacle to an honest closure of a person's life.

Beyond the Issue of "Truth=Telling"

Acknowledgment of the truth regarding a terminal illness is just the beginning; it is not simply a matter of "the truth, the whole truth and nothing but the truth." Supposing that one needs only to be forthright is an oversimplification. Blatant honesty can also be a serious violation of the personhood of the patient. An understanding of each patient, of his strengths and resources, ought to provide the basis of the doctor's decision about the best way to disclose information.

Today, the diagnosis of cancer no longer means an automatic death sentence; at least one third of all cases are successfully controlled or cured. Even in those instances where death is likely, there is a significant difference between saying to a patient, "You have cancer; there is nothing more we can do for you," and explaining what is physically wrong, describing the kind of care that will be given. Essential to any healthy acknowledgment of the truth is the assurance of continued medical support. If a patient is assured of good care, the ability to handle the reality of the illness is strengthened.

The quality of hope is not limited to medical definition. What may be considered medically hopeless need not be without hope for the human spirit.* A person with a terminal illness may hope initially that the doctors are mistaken; then, for cure or at least for treatment and prolongation of life. As the disease progresses, goals and expectations are altered and one lives for the realization of shorter-range goals—the completion of a thesis, the graduation of a child—and for everyday joys, such as the chance to see a special person once again or to watch another

*These ideas were presented by Elisabeth Kübler-Ross, Workshop on Death and Dying, Yokefellow Institute, Richmond, Indiana, July 1973.

sunrise. Then there is the hope that it will be an easy death, that one will not be forgotten, that the kids will be okay, that one will see God.

Our goal-oriented culture trains us to define the primary purpose of treatment and rehabilitation as the return of the patient as a functioning member of society. Not all patients, however, get better and go home. How does one interact appropriately with those patients for whom the traditional definitions of recovery and rehabilitation are no longer viable objectives? When one can no longer help a patient to get better, what can one do for that person? What *are* the alternatives to abandonment?

There are no guaranteed formulas for relating to a person who has a terminal illness. We have become so task-oriented in this society of ours that we may need to be reminded that it can be as important to "be" as to "do," to be present to the patient, even without words or actions. What, finally, can you really ever say to someone who is dying, except that you care about him and will try to be with him.

One needs to listen to the patient and take cues from his feelings. A theorizing or overanalyzing approach should be avoided. The patient may be experiencing any of a variety of responses, some of which may be quite unrelated to the fact that the illness is terminal—the food may really be awful, or the room too hot, or the bedpan still under him!

Elisabeth Kübler-Ross' descriptions of patient responses to terminal illness (denial, anger, bargaining, depression, acceptance) are very useful. I asked Mark once if he had any sense of moving through the stages that Dr. Kübler-Ross described. He replied, "Yes, many times over." There is no lock-step progression from denial to acceptance. One is not simply angry at one point and then never angry again. You cannot pull a patient kicking and screaming from stage one to stage five. You can only be present where the patient is at that moment, and you won't know where that is unless you are listening. If you're the one doing all the talking, you're not learning anything.

Sometimes patients reveal their feelings about their illness indirectly, through nonverbal language (artwork) or symbolic language (the description of dreams or twilight imagery). Sometimes a patient can find an opening to share feelings when a family member or nurse says, "Is there anything I can do?" or "It's tough, isn't it?" or "Do you want to talk about it?" I know an elderly gentleman who was surrounded by devoted family who refused to acknowledge that he was dying. He said nothing himself until a niece from out of town had a few moments alone with him. When she said, "Is there anything I can do for you?" he started to weep and said, "Just help my wife find a home."

The way a person addresses his own dying is very personal, and the person with whom the patient chooses to do that sharing will vary. It may not, in fact, be the person who offers himself up most readily for that purpose; one should not be offended by a patient's choice.

One family, who were eager to share everything openly with the mother, who was in the final stages of an illness, did everything possible to get her to talk about her dying with them. She ignored all of their signals. Finally, she asked to see an old family friend, a priest. The family made arrangements to bring him across the country to her bedside. The two of them had a pleasant talk together, and the visit ended, no mention having been made by her of her illness or imminent death. It was finally clear to the family that the mother neither needed nor chose to talk about her dying, that it was their own need to speak of it that they were experiencing. It is important not to project onto the patient our own agenda for sharing. We cannot help another with his or her own dying until we have come to terms with it ourselves.

Nor should we project onto another the manner in which that person should do that dying. Perhaps we have placed too much emphasis on helping the patient reach the "acceptance" stage. For some, there may be indignity in the very concept of death with dignity. For those who see death as the ultimate outrage, the most consistent, honest approach to the dying itself may be raging, a refusal to "go gentle into that dark night." Each person, finally, is in charge of his or her own response to that exiting.

It would be difficult for anyone, regardless of the degree of caring, to respond adequately to all the needs of the terminally ill person with whom he or she may come into contact, and one needs to acknowledge that limitation in one's own energy and availability. There will always be some patients with whom there does not exist the necessary or appropriate rapport, and it is important to acknowledge that limitation as well.

The real burden of addressing terminal illness openly is that openness can be abused by jargon, by setting apart the person who is ill. The risk of identifying the needs of the terminal patient is that we may lose the person in the process of categorizing, so that the person with a malignancy is seen as having *only* a malignancy and no other qualities. A student researching a paper on thanatology walked into a patient's room and asked, "And how are you feeling about your dying today?" It is the task of everyone—family, friends and medical professionals—to help that person to *live* until he or she dies.

Health-care professionals are frequently taught that personal involvement with patients threatens objectivity and competence. There are undoubtedly instances when this is so. No one should be asked to work nonstop on a burn ward or intensive-care unit. One cannot give emotionally and physically of one's self for an extended period of time without cost to one's own emotional energy.

Perhaps there would not be such a need for professional distance if medical institutions provided outlets for defusing the strain which such involvement entails. Those who work most closely with patients who are critically ill (i.e., the nurses who are with such patients around the clock, not just during the early morning grand rounds), ought to have a supportive community within which to proceed. There should be built-in opportunities for revealing feelings and frustrations, in-service workshops, and discussions of the best procedures of caring for a patient as the disease takes its course. Medical institutions should encourage their staff to reinforce and affirm each other's efforts so that nurses and physicians need not feel alone in their attempts to care for a patient who is facing death—a death which, as members of the helping profession, they face as well.

4

Living in a "Meanwhile"

How does one proceed in a "meanwhile"? When you can no longer assume recovery, how do you face the future? The time of remission, therapy and subsequent hospitalizations is filled with both anxiety and hope; it is a time of tension and adjustment for family members and patient alike. Family difficulties often are exacerbated, and everyone must make a special effort to understand the other's feelings.

There are specific fears commonly associated with a critical illness. Awareness of their nature and origin may help the patient to deal with them more openly. In *Mother Anxiety and Death,* Joseph Rheingold sets forth the premise that man's deepest fear of death lies in the subconscious, in the fear of "a catastrophic force bearing down upon one over which one has no control."[1] The symbolic representation of this fear, in dream imagery or nonverbal artwork, may take the form of huge pillars towering over a small human figure or of an advancing tank or train. When people are asked to imagine their own death or the death of someone they love, they are more likely to use destructive, violent imagery than to envision death by aging or disease. Mr. Miller, in Robert Downs' novel, *Going Gently,* says, "Everyone thinks that when he gets it, it's going to be quick, splendid, and with just a dab of heroism. No one ever thinks he's going to be nibbled away."[2] Our fear of death is largely determined by our subconscious fear of the dying itself, the means by which we meet our death. The person with a terminal illness at least has the advantage of being able to identify the catastrophic force responsible for his end.

Fear of dying can lead to "continual, abject panic," and may be redirected or channeled into anger. "Soon you will be so angry that you will not even recognize yourself."[3] The release of that anger, however indiscriminately vented, can be cathartic. If families and staff know the source of the emotion, they can be more understanding of what appear to be attacks on themselves, the quality of their work or their efforts to please the patient.

In addition to the subconscious fear of death, there are a variety of conscious fears[4] that can often be relieved if addressed openly by the patient and those involved in his or her care. The fear of abandonment is probably the patient's primary concern. Fear also arises, however, from not having adequate information with which to assess one's situation. Awareness of the progression and ramifications of the disease, of the purpose and effects of courses of treatment, can allow time to prepare for and cooperate with the "knowns." If patient and family are told, for example, that certain drugs often cause vomiting, loss of hair, lumps on the neck, depression or erratic personality changes, they will be better able to adjust to those effects on their lives. Patients are frightened by their own ignorance about their illness. Old wives' tales, other people's experiences, their own assumptions about their bodies generate fears that a sensitive medical person could allay by identifying and discarding the false information the patient himself brings to the crisis.

One fear is that of disfigurement and disability. The possible loss of a body part is a tremendous concern and often keeps patients from seeking treatment when it is most crucial. There is also concern about the physical disabilities that may accompany the downward course of an illness: incontinence, inability to feed oneself, loss of mobility or sensory loss. Doctor and patient should discuss these matters openly. The patient should participate in any decision to have surgery. Talking with someone who has had a similar experience can help lay the groundwork for emotional recovery. This can often be arranged through the hospital's social service department.

Feelings themselves may be a cause of anxiety for the patient. To lose composure or break down can be very threatening to one's self-image, especially if the sharing of feelings does not come easily or if tears have been traditionally considered childish or unmanly. We must give each other permission to cry, to move through the tears to a deeper sense of knowing each other.

Fear of pain, and anxiety about the ability to tolerate it, is another area of concern. Patients can be reassured by being told of the various ways to alleviate pain. A related matter is the fear of drug dependency, a significant concern for many patients if the illness is prolonged. Regardless of one's personal abhorrence of chemical dependency, drugs may be the only means by which one is able to function at all. The escalation of drug usage and the undesirable side-effects should be discussed openly between physician and patient. The patient must determine for himself the level of pain that can be tolerated. When Mr. Miller in *Going Gently* rejects a dose of morphine, the nurse advises him to be realistic. He replies, "That's precisely my intention. I am not going to leave this pathos-strewn life with my soul mortgaged to morphine. I shall go out observing."[5] On the other hand, if a patient wishes to be pain-free, that should be his right as well.

Another fear, especially at the time of hospitalization, is that of loss of control over one's own affairs. To submit to the hospital regimen, even when it is for one's own good, is no easy thing. The tone in which hospital procedures are carried out can help to ease the sense of rigid authoritarianism, the "we/they" dichotomy. Wherever possible, health-care professionals should involve the patient in personal decision-making, whether it be for such a simple thing as time for a bath or a consultation about further health procedures.

Patients themselves must assert their rights to participate in decisions regarding themselves. The hospital form granting unilateral permission for operative procedures needs to be examined closely. If, for example, you do not wish the surgeon to perform a radical mastectomy while you are still anesthetized for a breast biopsy, then do not sign the form as written. Cross out and rewrite the conditions of your consent. Control is often forfeited because of ignorance about the alternatives or because people don't want to be difficult or are simply overwhelmed by the situation. Ask, check and double-check.

When the disease goes into remission and the patient leaves the hospital, new problems often arise. There is a difference between having a terminal illness and actually dying. It is important for the patient to find an acceptable balance between realistic hope and preparedness for the worst. It is equally important for others to treat the patient as a whole person, not just as someone who is about to die.

Major role changes are often involved when a serious illness occurs in a family. Not being able to "mother" or to run a household as one used to can be deeply troubling. To have others caring for your children, making the meatloaf, folding the laundry differently, can be a demoralizing invasion of territory and threatening to one's self-esteem. Resentment builds, and the patient often strikes out at the very people who are trying to be helpful.

Sometimes the anger is quite justified. By being unconsciously patronizing in their attempts to help, friends and family can reinforce the patient's sense of disability. Real caring may mean resisting the impulse to help and instead encouraging the patient to do what he can for himself. The best action may be to stand back and wait to be asked, to tolerate the patient's struggle to do something independently, because the struggle itself is a part of the reclaiming of life.

If it is the breadwinner of the family who is ill, the family may undergo an upheaval in economic roles, not an easy adjustment for the former "head of household." If the patient in remission is able to work, the nature of the employment may need to change. Yet our society has trouble with people in remission. Those who must seek new employment are often considered bad risks by businesses that fear being saddled with long-term disability payments. Many resist employing a person who will only be able to work part-time. It is essentially a civil rights issue, especially for those "patients" who are considered medically recovered from a localized form of cancer. The American Cancer Society and Civil Liberties Union have taken up their defense in several cases.

Socially there can be problems too. Relationships with friends and colleagues often become strained and awkward: the healthy do not wish to be reminded of mortality; it is as if mortality itself were somehow contagious. People are frequently made uncomfortable by the obvious physical effects of the illness. Yet the distinction between having a terminal illness and facing imminent death needs to be recognized so that it is a person's life that is lived rather than just a death that is waited out.

Family role changes may also be strained and uncomfortable. There is a sadness and peculiar sense of loss that accompanies the need to "parent" one's own parent. Helping a parent, or even a spouse, to bathe or use a bedpan may cut across traditional lines of privacy. Such tasks need to be approached with a special tendering of the other—and a bit of humor whenever possible.

To feel, or to imagine yourself, a burden to others, even if they willingly accept that responsibility, becomes an additional frustration. The patient feels guilty, on the one hand, for being such a responsibility, and irritated, on the other, because the need for care is itself an affront, a denial of well-being.

The knowledge that one is terminally ill is a burden no one else can really share. In spite of everything a spouse or friends or children try to do, their very vitality and ability to give only compound the frustration. Those who have always been closest are the persons that the patient lashes out at now, driving them away even while knowing that he needs them more than ever.

Mood changes—from cheerful coping to deep depression—trouble both the patient and those who are around him. It may be a particularly difficult time for husbands and wives, as they are baffled and hurt by the unpredictability of someone whom they thought they knew so well.* The spouse with the illness may very well resent the life that is so obviously continuing for the other. The very vibrancy, sexual attractiveness and ability to cope (pay the bills, mow the lawn, care for the children) may be reminders of his or her own limited energy and time. An almost inevitable distancing occurs, even within the most intimate of marriage relationships. The living and the dying often feel out of phase with each other, their past intimacy interrupted by something which is finally unsharable.

A person who is ill often places unusually high expectations on certain occasions, anticipating or even demanding that *that* Christmas, *that* Mother's Day or *that* visit be perfect, since it might be the last.

Some family members may feel guilty for having failed to understand the patient better in the past. There can be new perceptions and sadness for past judgments. One is aware now of lost opportunities and the knowledge of finiteness may make the time left awkward and confusing.

This period of the "meanwhile" can be particularly difficult for children. They may be expected to devote more attention than usual to the family member who is sick, yet their understanding of the seriousness of the illness is tempered by their own vitality, and they are least likely

*Free Fall, by JoAnn Kelley Smith, Judson Press, Valley Forge, 1975, is a helpful personal account of these issues.

to be successfully manipulated or coerced into insincere behavior. They often bear the brunt of adult tension. Unattended, small children easily get into trouble, often injuring themselves. Incidence of accidental poisoning and falls increases during times of family crisis. If it is a sibling who is seriously ill, the other children often fail to understand the attention lavished on the sick child. Even understanding it, they may resent it. Children are often excluded from an understanding of the truth which might help them cope with that stress.

If parents are unavailable, adult friends can offer outings or piggy-back rides or the chance to make cookies. A comment such as "It's hard when big people are sad or worried, isn't it?" can provide an opening for children to speak up about their own feelings. Reading aloud books that deal with serious illness or loss is one way of preparing children.

Another source of tension is the anguish of seeing a loved one in pain, and the inability to mitigate that suffering. One's own grieving can inhibit ministering to the patient. A more impartial person, such as a compassionate nurse, often serves as a valuable presence at such a time.

Attending to the needs of a sick person can be tremendously draining, and it is not unusual for family members to wish it were all over, for their own sake as well as the patient's. The illness may become the pervasive dynamic in the family's life, the normal flow of a day disoriented by hospital visits, trips to the pharmacy, sickroom needs. Each day that remains is also a day of life. The terminal illness is not the only thing that is happening, either to the patient or to the rest of the family. However much we may care about another, it is important not to *all* be dying.

Another issue that arises during a terminal illness is the need for help from outside the family. It is not easy to relinquish control of one's own affairs, to let someone else rearrange your refrigerator or take your child to the school play. Most middle-class Americans have traditionally valued the notions of independence and self-reliance. We are programmed to manage on our own and feel ashamed at having to admit to others that our own resources are inadequate. We find it difficult to receive graciously what cannot be paid back in kind.

Yet we do need the help of others, particularly in times of crisis. Life does not require that we rise to every occasion by ourselves. We are essentially interdependent creatures, and our relationships are the less rich, the less whole, if we deny this. To admit it is paradoxically liberating. One is released from having to be brave or strong or capable all the time. It often happens that saying yes to a gift offered is a gift itself in return. To allow others to help acknowledges and affirms their connectiveness, their place as family or friends.

There are many ways that one can offer to help. People still need to eat, the lawn still needs to be mowed, the dog walked. Whenever I hear of someone else's bad news, I head for the kitchen. Up to my elbows in flour, it is easier to feel that I am doing something helpful. The offering of food has traditionally been a way of giving comfort—warm milk in the night for a child's bad dream—of ministering to a pain that is essentially untouchable.

"Let me know if there's anything I can do" is sometimes a way of saying goodbye—the offer itself taking care of the guilt while minimizing the risk of any real involvement. If you really want to help, think of something specific that you can do, and offer that. Vicki called the day after Mark first went into the hospital and said, "May I take care of Robin for you today?" Some who only said, "Do let me know," I never got back to—partly because it took too much energy to suggest just how they could be helpful. One tries to use one's resources and the offerings of others without becoming either drained or manipulative. The support and caring at the initial point of a crisis peaks and then drops off rapidly as time goes on. When a happy ending is neither imminent nor likely, hospital visiting becomes tiresome; requests for assistance, wearing and bothersome. The glow of charitable goodness wanes once the casserole dish has been returned. It's not easy to be the bearer, again, of bad news —to have to say, "Mark's back in the hospital, could you . . ." How do you call again for help when you imagine the friend thinking, "Oh, no, it's her again"? Yet the need all too often does continue. The real test of friendship lies in unglamorous giving and in being alert to this dilemma of recurring need. If those who care are aware of the awkwardness of having to ask yet again, then those who seek to help can offer first. What is needed is a support community, where the sharing of tasks can be spread among a number of friends.

Even when one is most in need of outside help, problems can arise. The very logistics of handling expressions of concern can be overwhelming: where to house visitors? what to do with three offerings of lasagna at the same time? Having someone to keep track of phone messages and dishes is a great help, while someone else within a church or neighborhood group can receive messages and answer questions which need not be addressed to the family directly.

Some people need to be needed beyond one's ability to respond. There are often times when it is easier to do something oneself rather than explain to another all the "how-to's." It's good to have friends to whom one can say, "Thanks anyway," and still know that they can be counted on another time.

It may be difficult for people who come bringing their own agenda about "the problem" to find the family in a different space emotionally from themselves. The outsider may be able to focus only on the terminal illness, while patient and family cannot respond in depth to the crisis all the time. Those who live with the disease and the prognosis every day may appear "strong" and "holding up remarkably" simply because that is the only way to get to the next day at all.

To be concerned with your own feelings when visiting someone with a terminal illness is to be conscious of only half of the relationship. Think rather about the person being visited. A visitor's anxieties about the implications of a terminal illness are nothing compared with what the patient has already suffered. He may need something as simple as the assurance that he is still physically acceptable. Lay awkwardness aside and direct your attention to the person you have come to be with.

During a meanwhile, perceptions of time and accomplishments are altered. The patient measures time by the intervals between pain, by another's smile, by the moments it takes a child to reach the bedside. For the family, the passage of time is blurred by the attention given to the patient. Then, abruptly, one is brought up short, outraged by helplessness and the knowledge that despite all the arrangements for the care and recovery of that loved person, the disease has its own agenda, and one is reminded again of the fragility of this time and space together.

5
Little Deaths*

Any illness means at least a temporary laying aside of certain normal patterns within a family. We were to experience—Mark individually and all of us as a family—a variety of losses and endings as his illness progressed. Acknowledging those endings as they occurred—such as changes in appearance, the need to use a wheelchair, the end of sexual activity (though not of intimacy) and the termination of career plans—was one way of preparing for the final closures that death brings. Throughout our lives, we experience many "little deaths" that prepare us for the experience of death itself.

Transitions, and the endings inherent in them, occur throughout life —at times of significant age change (entering the teens, turning thirty, reaching "half a century"); change in work position or home (graduation, job loss, retirement, moving); change in physical being (disability —whether through accident, illness or aging) and change in relationships (between children and parents; friends, lovers and marriage partners). The responses and needs felt at the time of a "little death" are often similar to those felt at the time of a terminal illness or an actual physical death. Denial, fear, anger, guilt, self-pity, bargaining, depressions and acceptance can be as real a set of reactions for someone confronted with job loss, loss of hearing, or the end of a marriage as for a patient faced with an inoperable cancer.

The "deaths" we experience when we are still expected to get up the next morning can be the most difficult—when the losses have to be lived with and through. They can become "corpses" that we carry around

*Much of my understanding of this topic has come from conversations and workshops shared with Dr. Ruth Purtilo.

inside us, our "albatrosses," and they take their toll on our psychological health until they are laid to rest.

Whenever little deaths occur, they serve as "dry runs" on death itself. The closures that precede final physical death are endings over which we do have some control and some freedom, however. How we handle them and their effect on our lives can prepare us for loss that is permanent. Grieving is natural in all instances of loss, and if it is done appropriately, it will facilitate a more wholesome proceeding with life.

Regardless of the nature of the death, it is important to acknowledge the loss, to claim the reality of the closure, to say yes to that truth. Verbalizing the situation, sharing reactions with others, particularly with others who have had similiar experiences, helps one to address a loss, whether it be of a job, a stage in life, a relationship or a limb that's been amputated.

It is also important, however, to claim the uniqueness of that loss for oneself. To have someone say "I know just how you feel" offers little accuracy and less comfort. While others can be supportive, the loss is personal and must be met as such. There is a certain power, finally, in being able to acknowledge an experience as one's own.

In all instances of adversity, growth and strength come from confrontation with the dark spaces of that experience, not from avoidance. The search for some value or significance to it all is the growing edge of any experience of loss. Not that it is somehow better to have lost that leg or that job or to have ended that marriage. The meaning lies rather in the realization that even within painful experiences it is possible to mature and come to a deeper understanding of both the limitations and transcendence of the human condition. One is then able to move through and beyond that loss, that death, and proceed with life.

6
Putting Your House in Order

It is a curious fact that in our culture we are encouraged to plan for everything except death; we plan for vacations and babies and "the college of your choice"; yet the one event that is for certain, the end of our life, remains a difficult topic for us to deal with openly.

Putting one's house in order means examining those areas of life which have to do with being mortal. That "house" includes the people in one's life—all the relationships, commitments and tasks with which one is involved (the day-to-day responsibilities—care of children, work at the office, committee chairmanships, the first bass part in the community orchestra); the "things" for which one is responsible (possessions, financial and business affairs—the car insurance and mortgage payments); the goals toward which one is working and the dreams yet to be realized; and one's emotional and spiritual being.

Life will go on for others after your death, yet the quality of life for them will depend in part on the attention paid now to that "business." The following pages seek to address some of the practical details of putting those areas in order.

Statistics show that the average married woman in the United States experiences ten years of widowhood. Seven out of every ten men predecease their mates. Yet many couples put aside the notion that either one of them might die before the other, as if ignoring that possibility could keep it from happening.

Topics people must deal with include funeral arrangements and finances. Because such matters are rarely discussed while there is no need, many people, older women in particular, are forced to pick up the pieces alone, at a time which is already stress-filled.

The women's movement has helped put more women in touch with the economic, legal and business world in which they live, but many are still caught in role expectations, and there are whole areas of skills and responsibilities taken for granted as the territory of one or the other spouse. When it is the wife or mother who dies, the male may have an equally long list of tasks with which to become familiar. There is much about which we all still choose to remain ignorant (wills, estate laws, funeral options, pension benefits), because we are uncomfortable with the fact of our mortality which such knowledge forces us to face. Because life, including its hardships, goes on for others after your own has ended, it can be an act of love to look carefully, together, at what your death would mean for your family.

There are two areas of specific information which need to be covered: arrangements necessary at the time of death (i.e., funeral or memorial arrangements) and information regarding your estate for those who survive you (i.e., will, pension and insurance benefits, financial status).

The information for the first area should be kept up-to-date and placed where it is easily accessible and known to somebody else (not in your safe-deposit box, which becomes sealed upon your death). It should tell the location of your will (every copy of it), the number and location of the safe-deposit box and key, where essential personal papers are kept (birth and marriage certificates, information on previous marriages (such as date, place, children), documents on separation, divorce and adoption, citizenship, military service papers, Social Security card (the funeral director usually needs this number) and auto registration.

The letter should include funeral and burial instructions. If donation of one's body or organs to medical science has been arranged for, then the pertinent information should be included. (An important consideration is the need to proceed with organ transplant as quickly as possible after a donor's death.) Personal preferences regarding funeral arrangements should be set forth—cremation or burial? special music? pallbearers? open or closed casket? donation to a special fund in lieu of flowers? —as well as information regarding the place of burial or the scattering of cremated remains. These are all decisions which someone else will have to make if you do not. To be able to follow your wishes at such a time can be a great measure of comfort to those who must carry out those final plans.

Include data that you want in an obituary to help your family as they compose that notice of death and tribute to life. Include also a list of persons who should be notified immediately of your death. The names of several key relatives who could relay such information to other family members and the location of an address book may be a way of helping your family not to overlook more distant friends. The names, addresses and phone numbers of the professionals that assist you should be listed for the family to consult if necessary (attorney, accountant, banker, investment counselor; life, auto and casualty insurance agents; doctor, dentist).

The second area of information is the material your family will need to pick up the pieces of life as they proceed without you. (Try to imagine someone having to take over your desk or file cabinet tomorrow.) The executor of your estate will need to finish whatever business has been interrupted by your death. Your family should know what your plans are if they are to function as you intended. To determine the benefits they are entitled to, they should know the names, numbers and location of your life insurance, medical disability and accident insurance policies. Your family will need information on all your cash and charge-card accounts, military service records, fraternal or religious organization affiliations, and your employment records, past and present, especially if your death is at all work-related. They will need to know where to locate your tax returns, what real estate holdings, securities or trust funds you may have in your name, and what debts may be owed to or by you. If you have made mortgage insurance arrangements to protect your home in the event of your death, your family should know where to find proof of such a transaction. (Insurance for waivers of debt on house mortgage or student loans is usually obtainable for a nominal fee, and can provide an important source of security for your family later.)

If these matters have always been your sole responsibility, inform your spouse or another family member now, while you are still around to share your insight and experience. If the intent of investments, insurance policies and home ownership is for the well-being of others besides yourself, then work together now on understanding those mutual business affairs. Help the person designated as the executor of your estate to be familiar with the management of your home or family finances, or at least informed enough to interact comfortably with the professionals to whom you turn. In the most loving of families, ignorance of these matters has caused avoidable hardship for the survivors.

Data regarding last things should be reviewed periodically and kept consistent with one's present situation. One should realize, however, that in spite of any amount of planning, the nature and place of death itself may require different arrangements from those determined ahead of time. What we can do for our families is to let them know what our preferences would be and then free them to do what is most necessary and appropriate when the time comes.

Helpful forms for compiling such data are available through the Continental Association of Funeral and Memorial Societies, Inc., "Putting My House in Order" Checklists, 1828 L Street, N.W., Washington, D.C. 20036, and *Teaching Your Wife How to Be a Widow*, a U.S. News and World Report Book, Appendix IV, "Checklist of Family Affairs" (1973), pp. 275–288. Formidable as it may appear at first, keeping such information complete and up-to-date can be an important act of caring for your family.

Far less complicated, yet also important, are items of personal property one may wish to give to others. It can be a very satisfying action —affirming one's part in the process of using and caring for special things and passing them on to others as a remembrance.

One's house includes personal relationships as well. The possibility of loss reminds us that we do not have forever to let people know what they mean to us, to work out differences with those we care about. One exercise used in Death and Dying workshops asks the participants to imagine lying in their coffin while family and friends walk past. All that one might wish to say or do at that point is "unfinished business," the part of one's house not in order. For those in the workshop, there is still time.

For most of us there will always be some business that remains unfinished: parts of the house in order, perhaps, but never finished. In spite of all the preparations, are we ever really ready to die? An eighty-year-old friend, his will made out and the insurance papers all arranged, starts to fall asleep these days and then jerks awake, acutely aware of his age and the real possibility of not waking at all some day. He gets up and wanders about the house, puts on favorite music, leafs through favorite books or stands at the window watching an apple tree by moon-

SHEAVES

142

light. Ready, but not ready; unafraid of death, but not yet willing to give up life.

Now I lay me down to sleep
I pray the Lord my soul to keep
If I should die before I wake . . .

> . . . that might be easier
> than living today
> knowing that having awakened before I died
> and seen life,
> I do not want to let it go.

—Ruth Purtilo

Not to know another spring,
The flowering of earth or child—
To fruit from blossom,
I to Thou—
O God, how?

—S.A.

7

Children with
Terminal Illness

The critical illness of a child must be one of the most difficult aspects of life and death that we are called upon to face. Yet even when we cannot assure a child that he will be better soon, there are ways to offer comfort.

Since even finger pricks for a blood sample can be interpreted as punishment for some unknown offense, young children need to be prepared ahead of time for the procedures involved in their treatment. They need to have some understanding of what is being done to their bodies and why. Play therapy and education* prior to treatment help to familiarize a child with the procedures of the hospital and allow him to participate more directly, calmly, in his own care. (By playing "doctor," the child is able to do to a doll what he most fears will be done to himself.)

Art and music can be valuable therapeutic tools for releasing emotions. The games children make up themselves, role-playing and story-telling, often reveal their concerns and questions, and can provide signals about the way they interpret the world around them.

One study done of anxiety in hospitalized children revealed that children with terminal illnesses who were thought to be unaware of their own prognoses registered anxiety twice as great as that of children hospitalized for other reasons.[1] Their drawings frequently depicted death. They were asked to make up stories about pictures they were shown, and 63 percent of the stories spoke of death. A majority of those children "ignorant" of the nature of their illness gave the characters in

---

*A good example is the Hospital Play Education program offered at Northwestern University and Children's Hospital.

the stories their own symptoms and diagnoses, spoke of loneliness, revealed fear, anger and anxiety about body integrity, assumed personal blame for their own illnesses, and expressed belief that their parents didn't care about them. One eight-year-old whose mother was determined that she should never be told the diagnosis concluded each of her stories with the death of the main character, angrily remarking, "And nobody cared, not even her mother."

Sensing the avoidance by adults of something too horrible to talk about, and fearful of losing whatever contact they still have, children keep silent themselves. "Protected" by adult silence, they are left to deal with their questions and fears alone, denied loving care where it is most needed.

With new medicine and methods of treatment, many once-fatal forms of cancer can now be arrested in young people. Yet even then, the emotional price is high. The stigma of having to wear a wig or stocking cap to school, the taunts of classmates and misunderstanding of adults can be devastating to a young person of any age, and often lead to a sense of failure and school dropout. "Learning to play the victim" as a result of attention derived from the illness may handicap a young person's development as a whole.[2] One solution lies in meeting with other children who are undergoing similar experiences.

Living with a life-threatening disease can be especially difficult for adolescents. At a time in life when a Saturday-night pimple has the import of a national calamity, treatment for basic physical survival often means rashes, nausea, vomiting, loss of hair or amputation.[3] The difficulty is compounded for teenagers when they are placed during treatment in pediatric wards, where the lights go out at 8:30 P.M., or in adult wards where many other patients are elderly persons in terminal stages of disease. Adolescent treatment centers, such as the Vincent T. Lombardi Cancer Research Center of Georgetown University, are needed to help young people deal with life-threatening illnesses in an environment where understanding among peers is possible.

As with adults, there is no pat formula, no recipe for response to the child who is dying. What one can do is give assurance that he will not be abandoned, that he is loved even in the most painful times. Perhaps it is because they find it difficult to conceive of nothingness or nonbeing that young people are not so anxious about the horizons which death has to offer. Life and death are equally uncharted adventures. Dying children have much to teach us about acceptance of our creatureliness and the potential of the human spirit.

8
Decent Terminal
Medical Care

Mark and our family experienced decent terminal medical care, an essential part of the "art of medicine." While the technology of medicine is oriented toward sustaining life and treating for recovery, the "art" of medicine requires an awareness of the whole process of human physical life, including its end. It means knowing when to stop the technology, when to "let go." Decent terminal care is the medical alternative to artificially maintained life, a course of action decided upon before the patient is hooked up to machines.

People who feel strongly about being allowed to die according to their own internal timetable should relate those feelings honestly to their physician and family. The "Living Will"* is a document that makes clear a person's wishes regarding terminal care. Such sharing ahead of time keeps the responsibility of decision-making focused on the patient.

When hope of recovery is no longer realistic or reasonable, it is then time for the patient, family and medical staff to acknowledge and set in motion a different order of priorities. It is the character not the quality of the care that should change focus. It is the time to waive typical patterns of hospital routine. It is no longer essential to take blood pressure or temperature readings at regularly scheduled intervals or to press patients to eat or consume a required quantity of fluids. It makes little difference to a person on the day of death if he has taken the proper pills, had a bowel movement or done the therapeutic exercises.

The focus of medical attention can be changed from rehabilitation and recovery to ensuring humane and dignified care until the end. This

---

*Published by Concern for Dying (formerly the Euthanasia Education Council) 215 W. 57th Street, New York, N.Y. 10019.

change is not always easy for those dedicated to the saving of life. The goal is now to keep the patient as comfortable as possible and to provide personal support.

Simple tasks that allow family members to participate in the care of the patient—giving a bath, helping change the bed, being included in the decision-making—all help to reduce their anguish and sense of uselessness. Families should not be made to hover silently in the background.

Visiting hours should now be waived or determined by patient and family needs. Most of us assume that the medical world knows best and do not easily challenge administrative regulations. Yet there are times when one knows clearly, as I did with Kim, that one's own priorities ought to supersede bureaucratic decision. Administrative policy does not, in fact, necessarily represent the position or feelings of the medical staff itself; rules and procedures are often just matters of unexamined long-standing policy. How much better it would be to require that children be accompanied by a responsible adult, and then, if necessary, make restrictions in cases of individual patients, rather than unilaterally to deny the benefits of young visitors to a patient's bedside. The emotional needs of the family as well as the patient need to be taken into consideration by institutions that claim to care for our well-being but treat only the physical problem. The task of carrying out decent terminal care should not rest on medical personnel alone. Patients and their families should make known their concerns and ask if certain procedures are possible.

Sometimes during the final stage of the illness, family members want a medical assessment of the possible time of death. They may be asking if there's time left to attend to a certain task, if someone a distance away should now be summoned. They may be asking whether they have time to leave for a bit, needing to know if the patient is likely to live until they get back. These questions always seem difficult for medical people to answer. Yet they are not being asked for a personal guarantee, but just an honest assessment of the medical facts as they know them. To answer such a question, medical people must be able to handle the concept of death itself—the fact that a patient is likely to die, even under their care, and soon. If the time left to a patient is faced honestly by all those involved, then medical knowledge can be used to reinforce and facilitate whatever strengths and resources of integrity the family might bring to bear on their own decision-making.

When the final stage of illness has been reached, it is the time for the medical staff to withdraw as much as possible and to permit family and close friends to be present. It is the time to arrange for the patient to have surroundings as private as possible, removed from the isolation of an intensive-care unit or the public aspects of a ward. It is inhumane for a patient to die alone in an ICU while loved ones wait outside for their five-minute-an-hour visiting allotment.

When death has finally occurred, the medical staff often continues to interact with the family, if only to ask permission for an autopsy. Concern for the emotional well-being of the survivors is essential if healthy patterns of grieving are to be encouraged. Sometimes the nurses and doctors themselves are directly touched by a patient's death, and space needs to be made for this. A "screaming room" has even been suggested, for staff as well as family, as an alternative to medicating and stifling emotional response.

Too often, however, family members are surrounded by an awkward, uncomfortable silence on the part of the staff, and they make a hurried, stunned retreat from an institution where only the business of recovery seems to be appropriate. Even simple gestures of concern—the offering of tea or the gathering together of chairs for the family members— provide a temporary compassionate setting in which the survivors can collect themselves and then proceed.

With all that is being written and talked about these days on the subject of death, it must still be remembered that we are dealing with one of the most mysterious and private experiences of the human per- sonality. While books and studies offer valuable insights into the process of dying, there is a certain presumptuousness about definitive statements or the categorizing of ways in which patients or family respond. When decent terminal medical care is provided, and the freedom and integrity of the patient are respected, then each individual orchestrates his or her own ending. Each death remains, finally, a deeply personal, separate and unique experience.

9

The Work of Grief

Give Sorrow words
The Grief that does not speak knits up
   the o'erwrought heart and bids it break.
      —*Macbeth*, Act IV, scene 3

Our culture has traditionally left the bereaved at the graveside. For those hours surrounding the public act, the immediate family and the community at large are given permission to mourn. We too often expect, however, that the funeral will take care of the business of grieving, and our sense of timing is skewed by our desire to get it over with.

He who lacks time to mourn, lacks time to mend.
    —Sir Henry Taylor, *Phillip Van Arlevelde,*
                 Act I, scene 5

As a social act, the funeral or memorial service serves to reaffirm the value of life—that of the deceased as well as those left behind. It provides the context for a community to deal with the reality of death.

But for those most acutely affected by the death, the funeral ceremony may meet only immediate emotional needs. If the death was unexpected, the family may still be in shock, unable to get in touch with their feelings until later. Yet the rituals of mourning end as the family leaves the cemetery. The approved forms of societal support are suddenly taken away, and the survivors are left to do the real work of grief alone.

The hardest time for many who experience loss occurs after the official funeral business is over. The lives of others are picked up where

they left off—the interruption, for them, only a temporary one. While
there is much that the survivor must learn to do alone, the sensitivity
of friends and family is needed now more than ever.

The "work of grief" has essentially two phases: acceptance of the loss,
and healing of the wound that loss has caused. Psychiatrist Eric Lindemann characterizes grief work as the process of "emancipation from
bondage to the deceased," "readjustment to an environment in which
the deceased is missing" and "formation of new relationships."[1] It is a
process which Edgar Jackson defines as "restoring interpsychic balance,"
"getting the self into equilibrium," "wholeness of being."[2]

Though we might be prepared for dramatic immediate reactions to
a death, we are often insensitive to the fact that there is a mourning
process that follows which is usually painful, lengthy and internal. As in
a case of severe frostbite, with the return of feeling comes pain. When
the shock itself diminishes, the survivors often experience active suffering, including physical distress and illness, and only gradual slow recovery. Physical and emotional changes are common. Dysfunction of the
nervous system, excessive sweating, rashes, poor muscle coordination,
shortness of breath, and, in some cases, even symptoms of the deceased's
illness may be experienced by a surviving family member.[3] Unexpected
emotional changes may occur—feelings of hostility and outbursts of
anger, indiscriminately directed. Statistics indicate that during the first
year of bereavement, the survivors account for the highest death rate of
any population group, due to suicide, accident or illness. They are a
"population at risk." Health-care professionals involved in the ongoing
care of a family can help prevent the destructive consequences of unresolved grief by contacting surviving family members and encouraging
an office visit or chance to talk.

It is characteristic of much of our culture to avoid or deny those things
that call forth sorrow. Our inability to confront terminal illnesses and
death honestly has been a measure of that avoidance in the past. Overt
expressions of grief are painful for others to witness. Most people in this
society live with unresolved sorrow of their own—"corpses" which they
carry around inside themselves—and they cannot easily support the
expression of sorrow in someone else.[4] Most of us usually choose not to
risk awkward silences or to expose ourselves to a sense of inadequacy
when facing another's pain. Unless it is choreographed within the

known patterns of a wake or calling hours, we are often unable to respond.

At a time of acute loss, being comforted is not enough. It is important for those in mourning to express the sorrow which is real and immediate, to admit how much it does hurt. Yet in much of our culture, emphasis is placed on the control of emotions, on keeping a stiff upper lip, and the person bereaved may feel pressure to keep feelings under control in order not to make others uncomfortable. Emotions are often suppressed because of expectations about oneself (Men don't cry), the need to maintain the morale of others (Don't cry, Mommy), responsibility for crucial tasks, lack of privacy or lack of understanding on the part of one's associates or peers.[5] It may be tempting, and all too easy, to so submerge oneself in career or study or children that one fails to attend to the grief work at hand. The dark spaces in our lives need to be addressed, however, not boarded up by means of a busy schedule. Either overreaction or underreaction to a significant loss may signal a need for help in working through and resolving the grief.

Those persons help most who are able to hear the feelings of another, who do not need to brightly change the subject at the first sign of tears, and who are not embarrassed to share their own feelings of loss. They help most who can be present with an unrehearsed agenda—who risk coming, even not knowing what to say.

Although the bereaved does not need to hear how bad someone else feels, the acknowledgment of a shared loss means a great deal. Those written messages which were the most helpful to me were from persons who shared their own emotions, who affirmed the life of Mark as they had known it, and affirmed me.

> I'm wondering if you remember the first night I met you and Mark. You were going to a Christmas party for his department and had on that beautiful blue velvet dress you had made. Mark was so proud of you. He kept making a fuss over how beautiful you looked. It was neat to see him so blatantly, openly proud of you. You must have many special memories like that, and I can imagine how hard it is when those memories pop into your mind . . . We're so glad to have known him.
>
> —Sue Becker

. . . There is much I want to say and don't know how to. To say thank you for what you and Mark shared with us is inadequate because in some way you two have become a part of us and are reflected in our awareness of each other now and the preciousness of what we share. So although I really know you little, I feel a deep sense of communion and friendship . . .

—Sue Tobias

I hope that some of the bone-deep weariness is beginning to drain away . . . In between the spasms of grief and the tears you'll know now and then that the light still burns and that no darkness can ever put it out. Biblical truths like that get up and walk around on two legs after you've known someone like Mark!

—Oliver Powell

You know, after all this time, I still "see" Mark so often around here. It's always a black beard, walking or riding a bike, and I almost wave before I remember . . .

—Fritzi (two years later)

At the same time that the person bereaved may feel himself diminished, the person who has died is often remembered as better than he actually was. Although this is to be expected to some extent, the idealizing should not be overdone or prolonged. Negative feelings, resentment at the hassles with which one is now faced, hurts at tensions left unresolved, need to be faced. To be able to acknowledge the foibles and shortcomings of the person who has died can be a great relief. Honest "recall," coming to terms with the past, is important in order to face the future.

One is often haunted by the things left undone, the "if only's" which accompany a loss. Yet there will always be things left undone; that is part of the human condition. We can use whatever lessons have been learned to enrich relationships with those who are still present to us, still here for us to use time carefully with.

It is usually advised that one make no radical changes in one's life style for a year. That may not always be possible, although time should at least be allowed to consider the best alternatives. Each family's situation will vary.

Part of the work of grief is coming to terms with the "things" which the deceased has left behind—clothes, toys, papers, possessions. To live among these belongings as if the deceased person were still around to use them is as much a distortion of reality as the attempt to wipe out all evidence of that life. Although painful, confrontation with those belongings can be a time for claiming the good that has been known together.

The "rooms" that we carry around inside ourselves will not be cleaned or put in order by simply moving one's body to a different location or redecorating the house. Such change may indeed symbolize a new stage in one's life, but only if the emotional work of the heart and mind and spirit has been attended to as well.

10
The Interior Year

We wasters of sorrows!
How we stare away into sad endurance beyond them,
trying to foresee their end! Whereas they are
nothing else than our winter foliage, our sombre
evergreen, *one* of the seasons of our interior year,
. . . not only season . . . they are also place, settlement, camp,
soil, dwelling.[1]

—Rainer Maria Rilke, *Duino Elegies*

While twelve months in black dress may not be appropriate for most people today, there *is* business to be done in the work of grieving that takes the full cycle of an emotional and calendar year. "Grief is an appropriate response to a devastating situation . . . The healthy thing to do is to feel miserable for a while." Psychologist Roberta Tomes encourages persons to "forget the stiff upper lip." "Is it unfair to your family if you decide to be crazy for a year? Sure. That's life, and life is sometimes unfair. One of my missions is to educate the public to that."[2] The commitment to care for one another within the family structure should include not just crisis intervention but support after the crisis as well.

There are many "firsts" that those grieving need to travel through— the first Father's or Mother's Day without that family member, birthdays, anniversaries, Christmas, Passover. There are many moments as one moves through that first year, and later, when one is caught off-guard again, in seemingly quiet spaces, by the enormity of the loss— coming upon some forgotten article of clothing, familiar handwriting or an old toothbrush; the innocent question of a child or stranger:

"Where's your dad?" or "What does your husband do?" or "How many children do you have?"

Then, at the end of a year's cycle, just when things seem so much better, one often experiences an "anniversary reaction," an emotional response triggered by the date itself. Dates, the signal events on our personal calendars, are as important as we need them to be. Although the anniversary of a loved one's death will always have import to those most immediately involved, the effect of that remembering will eventually take on different character through the spiraling effect of time itself. I baked bread for Mark's memorial celebration, and a year later I baked bread again. But the next May I drank a glass of wine with Rob and Becky, and then went dancing.

It is the long-term needs of the person grieving which are usually inadequately addressed in our society. We grapple clumsily with the need for sustained, nurturing communities, and usually hand over to institutions and professionals those who are out of step with the pace of everyday life and emotions: the grief-stricken neighbor, the problem adolescent, the lonely recluse up the street—all those who would intrude on our already scattered time and energy.

Yet the person who is grieving needs to be included in the gatherings of others—not regarded as an awkward fifth, or avoided and silently pitied. Exclusion by others socially only compounds the sense of loss. When you miss the stimulation of conversation with someone of the opposite sex, it's nice to be invited to dinner not just when a friend's husband is out of town. You need friends who are able to remember the person you are missing most, who are able to say, "Wouldn't Mary have liked . . ." or "Remember when John . . ."

I used to find the hour of dusk the most difficult, when day is closing down and other families gather together, and was grateful for calls from Becky and other friends checking on my day. There were friends who called or whom I could call, to ask if we could bring our dinner over and all eat together.

When no one else cares about one's body, it's hard to put any energy or investment into it oneself—hard to put together an interesting meal when there's no one to appreciate the effort. Many nights that first year we were on our own, I resorted to "womb food," simple dishes of macaroni and warm milk.

The cause and timing of death will affect the nature of a family's grieving. If the death is unexpected, overt expressions of grief may be intense, while in those families where "anticipatory grief" has already taken place, such signs of mourning may not be apparent. If the illness has been prolonged and painful, relief that the suffering of the patient and the strain on the family are over may be the predominant emotions. All are valid responses.

Patterns of grieving will vary even within families. Each person experiences and expresses grief differently. Yet family tensions often arise because the various members are at different stages of their grief work. When it is a child who has died, parents may find themselves out of phase with each other, especially if one of the adults returns to a profession outside the home, while the other remains in the setting where the absence of the child is most acutely felt. Marital conflict and even separation are not uncommon during such times, and the parents may need help to understand what the other is experiencing, and find equally suitable outlets for their pain. Likewise, the possibility of remarriage for a surviving spouse may be a difficult issue for other family members. Each must grieve according to his or her own timetable. Those who stand outside the experience of loss must seek to be as nonjudgmental as possible, not imposing a regimen of "appropriate timing" onto someone else's pain.

Yet how does one keep from being tyrannized by the past? How does one avoid inappropriate, unhealthy grieving? When does self-absorption become extreme and all-consuming? The tragic consequence of overindulgent self-pity is often real abandonment by family and friends who can no longer bear the continuous flow of morose self-centeredness.

Suffering, ironically, offers its own form of security. The future is an unknown, fraught with dangers and risks, while the role of the griever is at least familiar. The widow image, living among the mementos and memories of the past, is an identity, a definition to cling to. Yet that grief is unhealthy which continues to choose the path of pain rather than working through it.

One device for getting some perspective on despair is to write about it, even if you have never written before. In simple diary or journal form —incomplete sentences, expletives, whatever—put down your feelings regularly. Record your day's anguish, and accomplishments, however small. The act of writing helps to externalize and diffuse the pain, and illuminate the present. Looking back at earlier entries will help you to identify those things which have changed and the advances you have made.

The journey out of grief is not a straight ascent, not some lock-step linear process where sorrow can be crossed off like tasks completed. For a while it may seem as if the same ground is being traveled over and over, the wound as raw and exposed, the loneliness and anguish as real as ever. Then the pattern becomes more like that of a spiral, where similar occasions, holidays, rememberings bring pain and sadness, but experienced at a less intense level. There are longer periods of quiet between. The days become not just a matter of coping, but filled with more and more pockets of gladness, self-confidence and hope. The initial panic of managing finances, children and home abates, as more alternatives and solutions become clear. The ache becomes less devastating, and one's mind is able to turn to topics other than death and one's own loss. The past finally stops overwhelming the present, and one can begin not only to hope for the future, but to be present in the moment, where one is.

Ironically, tragedy can mean a time of enrichment as well as of loss. Relationships are deepened, truths affirmed and a whole new range of possibilities opened up. You may have to learn to live with yourself, to learn to like yourself all over again, or maybe for the first time. A death in the family, whether spouse or child or parent, brings you abruptly to a new awareness of who you are, as an individual and a member of the community. It is fertile ground, this new soil, "interior season," and with careful nurturing, the harvest can be a time of deepened knowledge, authentic selfhood and new growth.

11
"Over Your Left Shoulder"
=Children and Death

> Ring around the rosies,
> Pocket full of posies,
> Ashes, ashes,
> We all fall down . . .

Children are aware of death much earlier in their lives than most adults realize. Studies have shown active interest, knowledge and concern about death among preschoolers. By the age of two, children can begin "to develop a concrete concept of death if adults help them to understand and integrate their observations."[1] Edgar Jackson points out that "Everyone faces the death of someone important to them on the average of once every six years."[2] One child out of every twenty faces the death of a parent during childhood,[3] and almost every child experiences the death of a pet, neighbor, friend or grandparent during the formative years of life.

Yet our society on the whole works to deny this reality. Toynbee has

I am grateful for insights and understanding gained through the work and writings of others while preparing this chapter, and recommend the following texts in particular for a more comprehensive understanding of this important subject:

Erna Furman: *A Child's Parent Dies—Studies in Childhood Bereavement*, Yale University Press, New Haven, Conn., 1974.

Edgar Jackson: *Telling a Child About Death*, Channel Press, New York, 1965.

Earl A. Grollman (ed.): *Explaining Death to Children*, Beacon Press, Boston, 1967.

Sara Bonnett Stein: *About Dying*, Walker, New York, 1974.

said of our death-denying culture: "Death is un-American, an affront to every citizen's inalienable right to life, liberty and the pursuit of happiness . . ." This is an illusion that we foster within ourselves and pass on to our children.

We need to help our children, while they are young, to develop a realistic understanding of death as they encounter it in their daily lives —wilted flowers, a dead bird or a skunk on the road. If we help them with the deaths that they meet in their early years, they will be better able to mourn appropriately when faced with a death within their family or among their friends.

To deny children an understanding of death as a part of the life cycle may distort their appreciation of the quality of life itself. Those young people who flirt with death ("chicken on the highway," Russian roulette, drug overdoses) may claim not to be afraid, yet often reveal an inadequate sense of life's value and little understanding of the finality of death.[4] An honest facing of the facts about death makes possible a healthy adjustment to that reality, rather than morbid curiosity and illusions of escape.

We can begin to do our business about death, about our own mortality, and help young people do theirs, at any time; we should not wait until we are faced with an immediate personal loss, our own dying or that of another. This need not be a morbid task, but one that is essentially life-affirming.

> Death is our eternal companion . . . It is always to our left, at an arm's length. An immense amount of pettiness is dropped . . . if you catch a glimpse of it . . .[5]
>
> —Carlos Castaneda, *Journey to Ixtlan*

The best time to talk to a child about death is when it is a part of the child's experience, when the child initiates the questions: "What is death?" "What makes things die?" "What happens to things after they die?" "Can it happen to my mommy and daddy? to me?"

Children learn much from our own responses as adults to the cycles of life, to loss and endings in simple as well as deeply personal things. They learn from our use or misuse of things; our concern or disregard for the resources of this earth (our ability to conceive of the *end* of things); our appreciation of natural beauty, though fragile. We can teach much through the cycle of seed to bloom and back to seed, the end of one life making possible the beginning of another.

When a pet dies or a dead animal is found, we can explain the difference between being asleep and dead. We can help them to express whatever feelings they may have (sadness, anger, guilt, disgust), and encourage the mourning process through burial rituals.

The attempt to come to terms with death and our own mortality is a lifelong process. No one of us understands death fully. All of our efforts to puzzle out its meaning for our lives need to be respected—the door left open for doubt, questions, differences of opinions, growth.[6] It is all the more so for young people. The answers that we give to their questions need to be ones that can be built on later—not ones that have to be discarded or unlearned because they were false to begin with.

No matter how well a parent explains things, a child will misunderstand some things, taking in what is most useful, what he most needs to hear at the moment.[7] Yet seed-thoughts can be planted, and they too are nurtured by time. If the channels of communication are kept open, then young people can share their confusions, anxieties and questions.

A Death in the Family

When a death occurs within a family, adults, out of a genuine desire to "protect" the child, often amend the truth by evasions and "doctoring" the facts. Explanations such as "Mommy has gone away on a long trip," however, may cause the child to wonder why Mommy has gone away without saying goodbye, and why she does not return. Religious explanations such as "Your Daddy was so good God wanted him to be in heaven with Him" or "Jesus came and took Baby away last night" may develop deep distrust and anger toward such a God and great ambivalence about the consequences of being "good." Our actions often contradict the words we offer for comfort.[8] If we tell a child only that "Gramma has gone to heaven," yet are inconsolable ourselves, it can increase confusion about what has really happened. Regardless of one's religious position or interpretation of an afterlife, it is important to help young people understand that a real ending of physical life has taken place. While it may be comforting for a child to be told that he'll see his daddy in heaven someday, it is essential that the physical death, the loss, now, be acknowledged. We need to respect the integrity of children. They will know if we are not being truthful or will find the truth out in other far more painful ways later. For many, deep roots of anger lie in having been so deceived as children.

At the time of the death itself, the simplest truth is usually sufficient. A child's response will indicate what more he or she needs to know just then. A child's questions are an expression of feelings, and need to be treated with respect. If the anxiety expressed in a question is evaded, the child may hesitate to express feelings openly, and remain caught in his or her own interpretation of reality. Those gaps in the truth not supplied by adults will be filled by means of a child's own fantasy.

As adults we need to try to hear the question that a child is really asking, and answer it as directly and honestly as possible. If you're not sure what it is the child wants to know, ask a question back before you answer (What do *you* think will happen when you die?). Try to respond simply. A lengthy discourse on the mortality of man or your personal eschatology is unnecessary. As time goes on, be alert for questions asked without question marks—for the statements that reveal misunderstanding ("When you go to the hospital for a long time, you die"). Be as honest as you can; if you don't know an answer, admit it. A child needs most to be able to trust those with whom he shares his feelings and questions, and to be reassured about the value and ongoingness of life —his own and that of other loved ones around him.

For children, as well as adults, the funeral can be an important time for sharing in a ritual which honors a life lived, acknowledges the reality of its end, and permits the expression of a shared grief. Young people may want to see the body of the person whom they have loved, to have a last chance to pat a grandfather's cheek or touch a hand. No ritual such as kissing the body should be forced on a child, however; each needs to say goodbye in his or her own way. Explain the procedure of a funeral or a visit to the funeral home ahead of time; ask the child if he wishes to be present, and then trust the answer. If a child who wishes to is not allowed to attend the funeral, he may interpret the exclusion to mean that his own feelings of sorrow are not worth sharing with others.

Helping Children to Mourn

Children, like adults, need time to mourn, and they need the understanding and help of those around them that they may do it fully. The intensity of mourning will vary, depending on the role of the deceased in the life of the child, the age and maturity level of the child, previous experiences and understanding of death, and the stresses experienced by the child surrounding the death. If the loss is immediate and personal, mourning occurs regardless of age. Once the stage of "object constancy" has been reached—for most children by the second half of their first year of life—the loss of that "love object" is known and felt.[9]

Various stages of children's understanding have been identified: death perceived as absence; as something mutilating or deforming, a threat to one's own body; as something that can happen to oneself and persons that one cares about; as a universal—a reality experienced finally by all living things. It is important not to categorize a child's level of understanding by age group, however; to assume that a child has no response to death, just because he or she hasn't yet reached a certain age. We might be comforted by imagining that a child is too young to know what's really happening, but it is faulty comfort.

For a child the task of mourning, especially if it is a parent who has died, will be significantly different from that of an adult. While adults usually have their emotional ties, love, energy, attention, invested in a variety of important relationships, a child's central focus is his or her parents. "Only in childhood can death deprive an individual of so much opportunity to love and be loved and face him with so difficult a task of adaptation."[10]

There is no prescribed "right" or "wrong" way to mourn the death of someone special. Each individual brings his or her own history, personality, resources, weaknesses and strengths to the difficult experience of loss. "Each step in assisting a bereaved person becomes valid only when it grows out of full acceptance of, and respect for, the feelings and facts that comprise the individual's personal situation."[11]

In order for a child to mourn adequately, he needs the assurance of continued care, to know that he is still important, his own life is still worth living, and that the other significant relationships in his life continue. A child needs to be assured that even if the adults around him are sad and preoccupied, they have not forgotten him and will recover, that whatever distress his family is experiencing, it is not so great that it negates their love for him.

While children ought not to be overwhelmed with frightening details or speculation about "how it happened," they do need to know what has happened, to be given solid facts to hold onto in order to allay the anxiety that the same thing is about to happen to themselves or other loved ones. They must feel that death is "not contagious . . . that others about them expect to live for a long time . . . At a time when a child experiences uncertainty, loss, insecurity and fear, he needs to be given information (where possible), closeness, warmth, evidence of adult calmness and confidence."[12]

Children can handle the truth, and the grieving of adults, in "pediatric doses." A parent's overt distress may be easier for them to deal with than controlled silence. Exposure to grief gives a child an important understanding of the reality of the situation. Seeing the intensity of feeling of others may help to validate the child's own feelings, confirm the importance and love felt for the person who has died, and reinforce a child's trust in the quality of the loving relationships which he participates in as well. ("If something happened to me, they'd feel bad then too.")

Children need to know that it's all right to have deep feelings of sorrow; to see adults cry, and be permitted the release of tears themselves. Grief shared within a caring environment facilitates the process of mourning and the journey toward healing.

At the same time, if possible, a child should be spared uncontrolled expressions of despair or complete collapse on the part of those adults upon whom he depends for emotional security.[13] If the adults in a household are too distressed themselves to answer questions, they can at least assure younger members of the family of their ongoing love and explain that they will be able to talk more about it all later. Expressions of grief need to be tempered in the presence of children by enough wisdom and maturity so that a child can trust that the adults about him are still able to function as dependable persons within his own world.

A surviving parent plays an essential part in assuring the child that the fabric of family life has not been totally destroyed. While it may be difficult, it is important that the parent not withdraw completely into a private grief, that the widow or widower continue to show responsibility and, over time, provide a model for working through the pain and finding worth in life once more.

The Task of Mourning

The task of mourning can be seen as fourfold: 1) understanding and accepting the concreteness of death, separating reality from fantasy; 2) expressing feelings and responses to the loss; 3) differentiating self from the person who has died; and 4) resuming one's emotional life and personal development.[14]

Understanding the Reality of Death

The task of mourning cannot begin until the reality of the death itself is acknowledged and believed. If we are to help young people complete their grief work, we must be sure it is possible for them to begin it. "Only straightforwardness gives a child the internal strength to deal with things, not as they imagine them to be, but as they are."[15] Children need to know the real reasons for the death in order to know that it is not their fault. (Too often careless expressions like "You'll be the death of me" or a child's fanciful wish that so-and-so would "drop dead" or "get lost" lead to great anguish and belief in personal responsibility for a death.)

Distinctions between fantasy and reality for children are still unclear. Human physical functions which end at death (moving, seeing, hearing) are often extended, magnified in children's imaginations so that the dead are perceived as an ever-present force, watching over and monitoring one's behavior on earth like a guilty conscience. Children may need help distinguishing between religious belief in immortality of the spirit, something which transcends our earthly life, and the concrete reality of physical death. Acknowledgment that the loss is permanent is necessary before the loss can be mourned, and the emotional ties to the deceased finally released. Part of the work of grief is giving up, letting go of the person who has died. Until that happens, one is not really freed to go on with life.

Expressing Feelings—Emotional Responses to Loss

Children will act out their grief in different ways. Some may withdraw into indifference or seeming apathy to protect themselves against emotions that are too strong for them to handle at the time. A child unable to cry at a huge loss may dissolve into tears over a broken shoelace or a lost doll. For many young children, aggressive or destructive behavior may be a way of testing the margins, checking out the perimeters of a world they thought they'd known, confirming the validity of a world thrown out of kilter by the loss.

Children's emotional response to loss often includes anger and guilt as well as sadness—anger at having been left, abandoned by someone whose presence they had counted on, guilt at having sometimes wished that person would die. Kids should be encouraged to express their feelings, to experience their own sadness, yet not be overwhelmed by it. Adults can help ease the guilt, anger and sadness by directing the release of those feelings through constructive channels, through physical activity as well as words—hammering, whanging tennis balls, painting, music. Opportunities can be offered, through small support groups in the classroom, church or wider community, for young people to talk with other kids who have experienced loss. If children are given permission and channels through which to express genuine feelings while they are young, they will be able to meet and respond with greater honesty and sensitivity to all of life's experiences, enriched by the capacity to be touched deeply by both joy and sorrow.

Differentiating Self from the Deceased—Healthy Identification and Remembering

A third aspect of the task of mourning is being clear about the separateness between oneself as mourner and the deceased. The fantasy that one is going to experience the same fate as one's spouse, older brother, parent—soon or at a comparable age—often causes a fearful imagining that can paralyze one's ability to finish the mourning process or go about living. Recognition of the concreteness of the other's death, real information about the cause of that specific death, as well as distinction between different kinds of death (old age, drunken hit-and-run, terminal illness, war) are important tools for separating the fate of the deceased from one's own present and one's future. Reassurance that one is not about to die oneself, that one does indeed have a chance to continue living, is necessary for the survivor to claim his or her own reality, to see value and meaning in taking up the threads of life again.

The process of remembering is one way to work through the anguish of grief, a way to defuse the sense of loss—not wistful longing for a future that cannot be, but laying claim to that which one has known.

It eases the missing to be able to talk of the person who has been special in one's life. Young people may need help in sharing those memories, consciously articulating the good that they have known in a relationship. Speaking easily, gently and a little at a time at first, about the person who has died, helps children to know that, as painful as the loss itself may be, it is not so devastating that it can't be talked about. They will have their own memories and need to be given the chance to clear up what they have not understood, and have validated what is true—to laugh over the funny parts, and cry over the sad. Talking about what happened in the past is one way of marking the boundaries of reality.[16] Distinguishing between what was real then and what is real now helps prevent fantasies from tyrannizing the present.

Ways need to be found for celebrating the importance of the person who has died and the effect she or he has had on one's life. The storying process—remembering those who have been a part of one's personal history—can help give young people a sense of rootedness and continuity, a way of acknowledging the loss, yet affirming the ongoing gifts of a life that has touched one's own. If the remembering is done fully and well, the difficult and ugly parts (images of the accident, things regretted, hurts unresolved), as well as the good, then that which has meaning and validity for the future can be kept, and the rest laid down, with deepened wisdom about what it means to be human, and a sense of grace.

While it is important to differentiate one's self and one's own fate from that of the deceased, some identification with the person who has died can be a healthy, integral part of the mourning process. Affirming the relationship between oneself and the person who has died, the ways in which one is still connected—similar physical characteristics (long eyelashes, slender fingers, smelly feet), personality traits (infectious laugh, way of standing), skills (artistic talent, musical ability, "a head for figures")—can help to ease the sense of loss for a child, reinforce self-image and integrate the past with the present constructively. Identification with the deceased that is natural and consistent with one's own self can be a healthy part of a young person's development, while that identification that is artificial and strained through anxiety or guilt at being still alive oneself (i.e., a younger child trying to duplicate the personality or achievements of a deceased sibling) needs to be redirected.

Each family has its own way of handling grief, and each response to loss is individual and unique. If the emotional burden becomes too much for a child to handle, however—if the hostility or withdrawal or sadness is unending; or if the external stresses are too great (hospitalization of the child or the surviving parent, loss of familiar environment, other family problems)—then counseling for family and child can provide help.

Sigmund Freud maintains that the principal task of mourning is "decathexis"—the withdrawing of all attachment to the loved object which no longer exists. "Reality testing proceeds to demand that all libido shall be withdrawn from its attachments to that object."[17] Yet Furman's work suggests that "mourning never does, nor necessarily should, succeed in the withdrawal of all investment."[18] For those most directly affected by a death, the sense of loss continues in some measure throughout life. Even when the mourning itself is finished, emotional and psychological connections are never completely severed. If it is a father or mother who has died, a child will deal with the absence of that parent at each major "signal" event of life (graduation, marriage, parenthood). A young person will continue to need information about that parent at each new stage of growth,[19] incorporating, or laying aside, what he learns—enlightened, stretched, enriched, by increased knowledge of family roots and influences as his own life and personality develop.

The final task of grief work is to complete the mourning process so that one is able to take up the threads of one's emotional life again, to pick up the pieces in such a way that one is freed to make new emotional commitments.

> I don't want to love her so much . . . I don't want to love anyone so much if they have to die . . .
>
> —A young woman as her mother lay dying

If the work of grieving is not completed, the bereaved person may cling to fantasies of the person who has died, afraid to care deeply about anyone else again, immersing self in memories or work or possessions.[20]

It is important to help children finish mourning so that they will be able to reinvest their love and energy and trust in other persons who share their lives. It often happens that a child is ready for a new parent before one is available, or is offered a new parent before he or she is ready. Sensitivity and patient understanding on the part of all the adults involved can help a child to accept new relationships while still honoring the feelings which he or she has for the person who has died.

The loss, as great as it may be for a young person, needs to be placed in perspective with the whole patterning of life. Children need to know, in spite of experiences of sadness and loss, that life is still worth living, that there is still much to take joy in, much to be loved; to learn not only that it is all right to cry, but that it is all right to laugh again as well.

12

Harvesting

Life carries death with it like a seed.

The gift of life is inseparably united to the promise of death; on no other terms is life ever given.[1]

—Bradford Smith, *Dear Gift of Life*

Recognition of our finiteness as human beings, our participation in a life cycle which includes our own death, is an essential condition of authentic selfhood. Not a nihilistic embrace of destruction, nor pietistic acquiescence. Neither revolt against nor evasion of death, but an openness to the reality of our finiteness—to the fear and the dread and the awesomeness of that mystery.

As the dark passages of a symphony are integral to the musical work as a whole, so ought we to own the dark places in our lives—pain, anguish, death—in order that we may claim the harmony as well.[2]

An authentic relationship to death is a touchstone of authenticity in all other relations.

—Heidegger

Acknowledging the impermanence, the fragility of any relationship, of life itself, sharpens awareness and appreciation of the time one does have. To see death as an integral part of the life process, to see oneself a part of a larger whole, to accept the certainty of one's own death, however and whenever it may occur, is to stand genuinely within that process. It frees one, finally, to taste more fully of life.

NOTES

CHAPTER 5

1. Bradford Smith, *Dear Gift of Life,* Pendle Hill Publications, Pamphlet #142, pp. 30–31.

CHAPTER 6

1. Smith, *Dear Gift of Life,* p. 12.
2. Elisabeth Kübler-Ross, *On Death and Dying,* Macmillan, New York, 1969, p. 87.

CHAPTER 7

1. John Woolman, *The Works of John Woolman,* T. E. Chapman, Philadelphia, 1837, *A Plea for the Poor,* Chapter 10, p. 342.

CHAPTER 8

1. Paul Tillich, *The Eternal Now,* Scribner's, New York, 1963, p. 35.
2. Margery Williams, *The Velveteen Rabbit,* Doubleday, New York, p. 17.

CHAPTER 9

1. Grollman, Earl A., *Talking About Death: A Dialogue Between Parent and Child,* Beacon, Boston, 1972 (new edition, 1976).

SHEAVES 4

1. Joseph Rheingold, *The Mother Anxiety and Death: The Catastrophic Death Complex,* Little, Brown, Boston, 1967.

2. Robert Downs, *Going Gently,* Bobbs-Merrill, New York, 1973, p. 28.
3. Ibid., p. 28.
4. Conscious fears—identified by William Worden, workshop lecturer, Lynnfield, Massachusetts, March 4, 1975.
5. Downs, *Going Gently,* p. 15.

SHEAVES 7

1. Eugenia H. Waechter, "Children's Awareness of Fatal Illness," *American Journal of Nursing,* June 1971, pp. 1168–1172.
2. Jean Dietz, "Stigma of Cancer," Boston *Globe,* September 13, 1978, p. 77.
3. B. D. Colon, "Cancer Treatment Center for Teenagers," Washington *Post,* December 23, 1976, p. 1.

SHEAVES 9

1. Erich Lindemann, M.D., "Symptomatology and Management of Acute Grief," *American Journal of Psychiatry,* September 1944, p. 143.
2. Edgar Jackson, workshop lecturer, Lynnfield, Massachusetts, February 1975.
3. Abby Stitt, R.N., "Emergency After Death: How Office Nurses Can Help," *Emergency Medicine,* March 1971, pp. 270–279.
4. Richard M. Magraw, "Grief—Its Clinical Importance and Its Resolution," *Modern Medicine,* May 29, 1972, pp. 61–65.
5. Ibid.

SHEAVES 10

1. Rainer Maria Rilke, *Duino Elegies,* translated by J. B. Leishman and Stephen Spender, Norton, New York, 1939, p. 79.
2. Roberta Tomes, Boston *Globe,* "Being Crazy for a Year Is Healthy," November 17, 1977, p. 2.

SHEAVES 11

1. Erna Furman, *A Child's Parent Dies,* Yale University Press, New Haven, Conn., 1974, p. 13.

2. Edgar Jackson, *Telling a Child About Death*, Channel Press, New York, 1965, p. 66.
3. Sara Bonnett Stein, *About Dying*, Walker, New York, 1974, p. 8.
4. Jackson, *Telling a Child*, p. 75.
5. Carlos Castaneda, *Journey to Ixtlan*, Touchstone, New York, 1972, pp. 54, 55.
6. Grollman, *Talking About Death*, p. 223.
7. Stein, *About Dying*, p. 5.
8. Elisabeth Kübler-Ross, Workshop on Death and Dying, Richmond, Indiana, July 1973.
9. Furman, *A Child's Parent Dies*, p. 43.
10. Ibid., p. 12.
11. Ibid., p. 11.
12. Jackson, *Telling a Child*, p. 72.
13. Ibid., p. 40.
14. Furman, *A Child's Parent Dies*, a composite of suggestions given in several chapters.
15. Stein, *About Dying*, p. 4.
16. Ibid., p. 22.
17. Sigmund Freud, *Mourning and Melancholia*, standard edition, Vol. 14, London, Hogarth, 1957, p. 244.
18. Furman, *A Child's Parent Dies*, p. 52.
19. Ibid., p. 24.
20. Grollman, *Talking About Death*, pp. 16–17.

SHEAVES 12

1. Smith, *Dear Gift of Life*, p. 16.
2. This was suggested to me by Deanna Edwards, Death and Dying Workshop, Richmond Indiana, 1973.

BIBLIOGRAPHY:

Books for Young People About Death

PRESCHOOL–FOURTH GRADE

Bartoli, Jennifer: *Nonna,* Harvey House, N.Y., 1975.

Borack, Barbara: *Someone Small,* Harper, N.Y., 1969.

Brown, Margaret: *The Dead Bird,* Young Scott, N.Y., 1938, 1965.

Carrick, Carol: *The Accident,* Seabury, N.Y., 1976.

Coburn, John: *Annie and the Sand Dobbies,* Seabury, N.Y., 1964.

Coutant, Helen: *The First Snow,* Knopf, N.Y., 1974.

DePaola, Tomie: *Nana Upstairs and Nana Downstairs,* Putnam, N.Y., 1973.

Dobrin, Arnold: *Scat,* Scholastic Book Services, N.Y., 1971.

Fassler, Joan: *My Grandpa Died Today,* Human Sciences Press, 1971.

Grollman, Earl: *Talking About Death: A Dialogue Between Parent & Child,* Beacon, Boston, 1973.

Harris, Audrey: *Why Did He Die,* Lerner Publications, Minneapolis, 1965.

Lee, Virginia: *The Magic Moth,* Seabury, N.Y., 1972.

Mathis, Sharon: *The Hundred Penny Box,* Viking, N.Y., 1975.

Miles, Miska: *Annie and the Old One,* Little, Brown, Boston, 1971.

Smith, Doris: *A Taste of Blackberries,* Crowell, N.Y., 1973.

Stevens, Carla: *Stories from a Snowy Meadow,* Seabury, N.Y., 1976.

Tobias, Tobi: *Petey,* Putnam, N.Y., 1978.

Viorst, Judith: *The Tenth Good Thing About Barney,* Atheneum, N.Y., 1971.

Warburg, Sandol: *Growing Time,* Houghton-Mifflin, Boston, 1969.

White, E. B.: *Charlotte's Web,* Harper, N.Y., 1952.

Zolotow, Charlotte: *My Grandson Lew,* Harper, N.Y., 1974.

Fifth Grade and Up

Armstrong, William H.: *Sounder*, Harper, N.Y., 1969.

Beckman, Gunnel: *Admission to the Feast*, Holt, Rinehart, N.Y., 1971.

Bond, Nancy: *The String in the Harp*, Atheneum, N.Y., 1976.

Buck, Pearl: *The Big Wave*, Scholastic Book Services, N.Y.

Burch, Robert: *Simon and the Game of Chance*, Viking, N.Y., 1970.

Carner, Charles: *Tawny*, Macmillan, N.Y., 1978.

Cleaver, Vera: *Grover*, J. P. Lippincott, Phila., 1970.

Cohen, Barbara: *Thank You, Jackie Robinson*, Lothrop, N.Y., 1974.

Commager, Evan: *Valentine*, Harper, N.Y., 1961.

Craven, Margaret: *I Heard the Owl Call My Name*, Doubleday, N.Y., 1973.

Donovan, John: *Wild in the World*, Harper, N.Y., 1971.

Farley, Carol: *The Garden Is Doing Fine*, Atheneum, N.Y., 1975.

Greene, Constance: *Beat the Turtle Drum*, Viking, N.Y., 1976.

Gunther, John: *Death Be Not Proud*, Harper, N.Y., 1949.

Hall, Lynn: *Shadows*, Follett, Chicago, 1977.

Hunt, Irene: *Up a Road Slowly*, Follett, Chicago, 1966.

Hunter, Mollie: *The Sound of Chariots*, Harper, N.Y., 1972.

Kaplan, Bess: *The Empty Chair*, Harper, N.Y., 1978.

Lee, Mildred: *Fog*, Seabury, N.Y., 1972.

Little, Jean: *Home from Far*, Little, Brown, Boston, 1965.

Mann, Peggy: *There Are Two Kinds of Terrible*, Doubleday, N.Y., 1977.

Moe, Barbara: *Pickles and Prunes*, McGraw-Hill, N.Y., 1976.

Morris, Jeannie: *Brian Piccolo: A Short Season*, Random House, N.Y., 1971.

Parks, Gordon: *The Learning Tree*, Harper, N.Y., 1973.

Paterson, Katherine: *Bridge to Terabithia*, Crowell, N.Y., 1977.

Peck, Richard: *Dreamland Lake*, Holt, Rinehart, N.Y., 1973.

Rock, Gail: *The Thanksgiving Treasure*, Knopf, N.Y., 1974.

Stolz, Mary: *The Edge of Next Year*, Harper, N.Y., 1974.

Whitehead, Ruth: *The Mother Tree*, Seabury, N.Y., 1971.

Windsor, Patricia: *The Summer Before*, Harper, N.Y., 1973.

Winthrop, Elizabeth: *Walking Away*, Harper, N.Y., 1973.

Young Adults

Guest, Judith: *Ordinary People*, Viking, N.Y., 1976.
Saroyan, William: *The Human Comedy*, Harcourt, N.Y., 1944.
Wilder, Thornton: *The Long Christmas Dinner*, Coward, 1931; *Our Town*, Harper, N.Y., 1960.

About the Author

SANDRA ALBERTSON lives in Concord, Mass., with her two children. She is a Quaker, studied ethics at Yale Divinity School, has led workshops designed to sensitize health professionals to the needs of the terminally ill and their families, and is currently teaching English part-time.